IMMUNOLOGY AND IMMUNE SYSTEM DISORDERS

THE FUNDAMENTALS OF HYPERSENSITIVITIES AND ALLERGIES

IMMUNOLOGY AND IMMUNE SYSTEM DISORDERS

Additional books and e-books in this series can be found on Nova's website under the Series tab.

IMMUNOLOGY AND IMMUNE SYSTEM DISORDERS

THE FUNDAMENTALS OF HYPERSENSITIVITIES AND ALLERGIES

MANZOOR AHMAD MIR
EDITOR

nova
Medicine & Health
New York

Library of Congress Cataloging-in-Publication Data

Names: Ahmad Mir, Manzoor, PhD, Department of Bioresources, School of Biological Sciences, University of Kashmir Srinagar J&K, India, Srinagar, Jammu and Kashmir, India, editor.
Title: The Fundamentals of Hypersensitivities and Allergies
Description: New York: Nova Science Publishers, [2019] | Series: Immunology and Immune System Disorders | Includes bibliographical references and index.
Identifiers: LCCN 2019957071 (print) | ISBN 9781536170122 (hardcover) |
ISBN 9781536170139 (adobe pdf)

Published by Nova Science Publishers, Inc. † New York

CONTENTS

PREFACE

Immunology is a distinctive subject that rose in the mid- 20th century. The subject developed as scientists started to unravel the mysteries about the defence system against pathogens. Researchers started to understand the mechanisms employed by the innate and the adaptive immune system in defence against pathogens. In recent years, the subject of immunology has been in prime focus as the various diseases that result in some immune-mediated disorders are caused by a failure of immune tolerance, that proves more detrimental than protective. Autoimmune Disorders like Psoriasis, still needs promising therapeutics and proper cure, for this a clear understanding regarding this one of a kind disease is very much needed. In the first edition of the book "The fundamentals of Hypersensitivity and Allergy" we have explained the Allergy, Hypersensitivities, their causes and types, underlying mechanisms of hypersensitivity reactions, various tests and use of them in diagnostics and therapeutics.

The book is organised into four volumes. The first volume comprises of ten chapters and it describe the rise, history and scope of immunology and the building blocks of the immune system *viz.,* cells, molecules and organs of the immune system. The chapter second describes the cells of the innate and the adaptive immune system and how the granulocytes and macrophages employ defence mechanisms to protect the body against pathogenic invasions. In the chapter third of this book, we have described the organs if the immune systems and how different organs are involved in the differentiation and maturation of immune cells. The chapter has also focussed on the structure of lymph nodes and their function in concentrating the antigens. In the chapter four of this book we have described the terms like antigens, immunogens, antigenicity, immunogenicity and how immunogenicity of an antigen is affected and how antigenicity of an immunogens is related to the immune response. The innate and adaptive immune systems and the different types of cells and molecules employed by the two branches of immunity have been described in a separate chapter. The structure and biology of immunoglobulins, their types and function in antigen binding and antibody dependent cellular cytotoxicity (ADCC) have been described well in chapter six. Focus has been laid on the distinction between and antibody and an immunoglobulin. The structure and function and major histocompatibility complex (MHC) has been described well in the book. The education of cells about self and non-self during their maturation and the processing and presentation of antigens by MHC bearing cells and how MHC coordinates both humoral and cell-mediated immune responses has been explained well throughout the book. The book has explained the complement system and its components, mechanisms and functions in a separate chapter. At the end of the book, we have given an insight about the vaccines, their history, development and how they are useful and helpful in the defence against diseases. The book also discusses the immune dysfunction and diseases associated with the dysregulation of immune responses.

The present book volume-4 entitled "The fundamentals of Hypersensitivity and Allergy" comprises of seven chapters and it describes the historical perspective, causes and classification of hypersensitivities, which are important in understanding the current issues regarding conditions in which the immune system which normally serves a protective role has a harmful effect. This book describes, the original concept of hypersensitivity and allergy and how the sensitive individuals respond to different allergens, drugs and other agents, where the body reacts with an exaggerated immune response, that ultimately results in tissue damage.

The classification of hypersensitive reactions given by Gell and Coombs with the modifications made to the previous classification are described well. Different types of hypersensitivities, their process, the contribution of various cells and molecules to normal immune responses and to hypersensitive reactions are described separately. The examples for different types immune responses are described thoroughly to get a proper understanding of the topic. The clinical manifestations of different types of hypersensitivities and their means of prevention, evaluation and management are also depicted with a clear insight are described in separate chapters. Lastly, the airborne allergens responsible for the allergy, different types of aeroallergens, their effects and allergies caused by them. The effect of climate change on aeroallergen production, various diagnostic tests for detection of aero-allergy with their prevention and control are discussed in detail separately. Various interesting and self-explanatory illustrations are incorporated to make the book useful to the students for whom it is written. The question bank which includes long answer type, short answer type and multiple choice questions with their answers at the very end of each chapter is developed to get a full grasp of the topic.

Dr. Manzoor Ahmad Mir

ACKNOWLEDGMENTS

Primarily, I want to thank Almighty for blessing me with his utmost grace and support. It was all by his grace that it was possible for me to accomplish my priorities.

There are some people to whom I am obliged and with whose direct or indirect efforts, it was possible to make this book entitled, "The fundamentals of Hypersensitivity and Allergy". Words are not enough to put my gratitude in, there are some great persons to whom I am really thankful and present my immense gratitude.

I am very grateful to express my feeling of immense gratitude and sincere respect to my mentors Prof Talat Ahmad, Dr. Javed N Agrewala, Prof Mohammad Afzal Zargar, Prof Raid Saleem Albaradie, Dr Abid Hamid Dar, Zahoor Ahmad Parry and Dr Nisar Ahmad Wani, with whose constant support, enormous patience, kindness, guidance and encouragement, I was able to reach to my destination. I have a huge respect for them and I admire them for the person they are. It was because of them that I became acquainted with the qualities they imprinted upon me through their knowledge and constructive criticism.

I owe deepest gratitude to my parents. A seed of loyalty, hard work, dedication and sincerity sown in me by my parents played a crucial role in completion of this work. They have been a source of great strength throughout my life. I would like to thank other family members for continuous and unconditional support of all my undertakings, scholastic and otherwise. Without their affection, support, best wishes, love and care this work would not have been completed

I would like to cordially thank Miss Najmu Nisa Research Scholar BGSBU for her support and co-operation. Mr. Aariz Manzoor Mir and Mr. Umar Mehraj deserves a special mention. I would like to thank everybody who was important to the successful realization of this book, as well as expressing my apology that I could not mention personally one by one.

Finally, I would like to thank again the Prime Mover Almighty in whom I have great faith

Dr. Manzoor Ahmad Mir

In: The Fundamentals of Hypersensitivities … ISBN: 978-1-53617-012-2
Editor: Manzoor Ahmad Mir

Chapter 1

HYPERSENSITIVITY REACTION

Manzoor Ahmad Mir*, Umar Mehraj, Safura Nisar, Bashir A. Sheikh, Syed Suhail and Hina Qayoom
Department of Bioresources, School of Biological Sciences,
University of Kashmir, Srinagar J&K, India

ABSTRACT

The term hypersensitivity arose from the clinical definition of immunity as “sensitivity” which is based on the observation that an individual who has been exposed to an antigen exhibits a detectable reaction or is “sensitive” to subsequent encounters with that antigen. Thus, hypersensitivity can be defined as a state of increased reactivity to a foreign agent usually acquired by a prior exposure to the same or a chemically related substance. Hypersensitivity reactions require a pre-sensitized state of host. Sensitization, or induction of the hypersensitive state, requires one or more than one exposure to the antigen, followed by a latent period. After the latent period, a reaction is elicited by another exposure to the antigen. The nature of hypersensitivity acquired is determined by the chemical composition of the allergen, the sensitizing route, the physiology and the anatomy of the host and other factors. The

* Corresponding Author’s Email: drmanzoor@kashmiruniversity.ac.in.

original concept of allergy included all immune-mediated diseases and the term allergy was interchangeable with the term "hypersensitivity." The term allergy was originally defined by Clemens Von Pirquet as "an altered capacity of the body to react to a foreign substance," which was an extremely broad definition that included all immunological reactions. Allergy is now defined in a much more restricted manner as "disease following a response by the immune system to an otherwise innocuous antigen." Allergy is one of a class of immune system responses that are termed hypersensitivity reactions. These are harmful immune responses that produce tissue injury and may cause serious disease. Almost every individual is allergic to some medium or the other in his/her lifetime. No human body is of the same composition and hence what could be allergic to someone can be harmless to another person.

Keywords: hypersensitivity, immediate hypersensitivity, delayed hypersensitivity, allergy, hay fever, allergic rhinitis, conjunctivitis

OBJECTIVES

- Define the concept of hypersensitivity
- Discuss the various causes leading to hypersensitivity
- Briefly describe various types of hypersensitivity
- To understand the phenomena of allergy
- Describe various types of allergies and their remedies

INTRODUCTION

An immune response mobilizes a battery of effector molecules that act to remove antigen by various mechanisms. Generally, these effector molecules induce a localized inflammatory response that eliminates antigen without extensively damaging the host's tissue. Under certain circumstances, however, this inflammatory response can have deleterious effects, resulting in significant tissue damage or even death.

This inappropriate immune response is termed as *hypersensitivity* or *allergy*. Although the word *hypersensitivity* implies an increased response, the response is not always heightened but may, instead, be an inappropriate immune response to an antigen. Hypersensitive reactions may develop in the course of either humoral or cell-mediated responses.

The ability of the immune system to respond inappropriately to antigenic challenge was recognized in the early twentieth century. Two French scientists, Paul Portier and Charles Richet, were the first to recognize and describe hypersensitivities. In the early twentieth century, as part of their studies of the responses of bathers in the Mediterranean to the stings of Portuguese man of war, jellyfish (*Physalia physalis*), they demonstrated that the toxic agent in the sting was a small protein. They reasoned that eliciting an antibody response that could neutralize the toxin may serve to protect the host.

Therefore, they injected low doses of the toxin into dogs to elicit an immune response, and followed with a booster injection a few weeks later. However, instead of generating a protective antibody response, the unfortunate dogs responded immediately to the second injection with vomiting, diarrhea, asphyxia, and death. Richet coined the term "*anaphylaxis*," derived from the Greek and translated loosely as "against protection" to describe this overreaction of the immune system, the first description of a hypersensitivity reaction. Richet was subsequently awarded the Nobel Prize in Physiology or Medicine in 1913.

With time, immunologists have learned that there are multiple types of hypersensitivity reactions. *Immediate hypersensitivity* reactions result in symptoms that manifest themselves within very short time periods after the immune stimulus, like those described above. Other types of hypersensitivity reactions take hours or days to manifest themselves, and are referred to as *delayed- type hypersensitivity* (DTH) reactions (Figure 1.1). In general, immediate hypersensitivity reactions result from antibody-antigen reactions, whereas DTH is caused by T-cell reactions.

As it became clear that different immune mechanisms give rise to distinct hypersensitivity reactions, two immunologists, P. G. H. Gell and R. R. A. Coombs, proposed a classification scheme to discriminate among the various types of hypersensitivity. *Type I hypersensitivity* reactions are mediated by IgE antibodies, and include many of the most common allergies to respiratory allergens, such as pollen and dust mites. *Type II hypersensitivity* reactions result from the binding of IgG or IgM to the surface of host cells, which are then destroyed by complement- or cell-mediated mechanisms. In *type III hypersensitivity* reactions, antigen-antibody complexes deposited on host cells induce complement fixation and an ensuing inflammatory response. *Type lV hypersensitivity* reactions result from inappropriate T-cell activation. It should be noted that, although this classification method has proven to be a useful analytical and descriptive tool, many clinical hypersensitivity disorders include molecular and cellular contributions from components belonging to more than one of these categories. The subdivisions are not as frequently evoked in real-world clinical settings as they once were.

The term *allergy* first appeared in the medical literature in 1906, when the pediatrician Clemens von Pirquet noted that the response to some antigens resulted in damage to the host, rather than in a protective response. Although most familiar respiratory allergies result from the generation of IgE antibodies toward the eliciting agent, and therefore are type I hypersensitivity reactions, other common reactions that are associated with allergy, such as the response to poison ivy, result from T-cell-mediated, type IV responses. With time, immunologists have learned that there are multiple types of hypersensitivity reactions. *Immediate hypersensitivity* reactions result in symptoms that manifest themselves within very short time periods after the immune stimulus, like those described above. Other types of hypersensitivity reactions take hours or days to manifest themselves, and are referred to as *d*elayed- *t*ype *h*ypersensitivity (DTH) reactions. In general, immediate hypersensitivity reactions result from antibody-antigen reactions, whereas DTH is caused by T-cell reactions.

We currently refer to anaphylactic reactions within the humoral branch initiated by antibody or antigen-antibody complexes as *immediate hypersensitivity,* because the symptoms are manifest within minutes or hours after a sensitized recipient encounters antigen. *Delayed-type hypersensitivity (DTH)* is so named in recognition of the delay of symptoms until days after exposure.

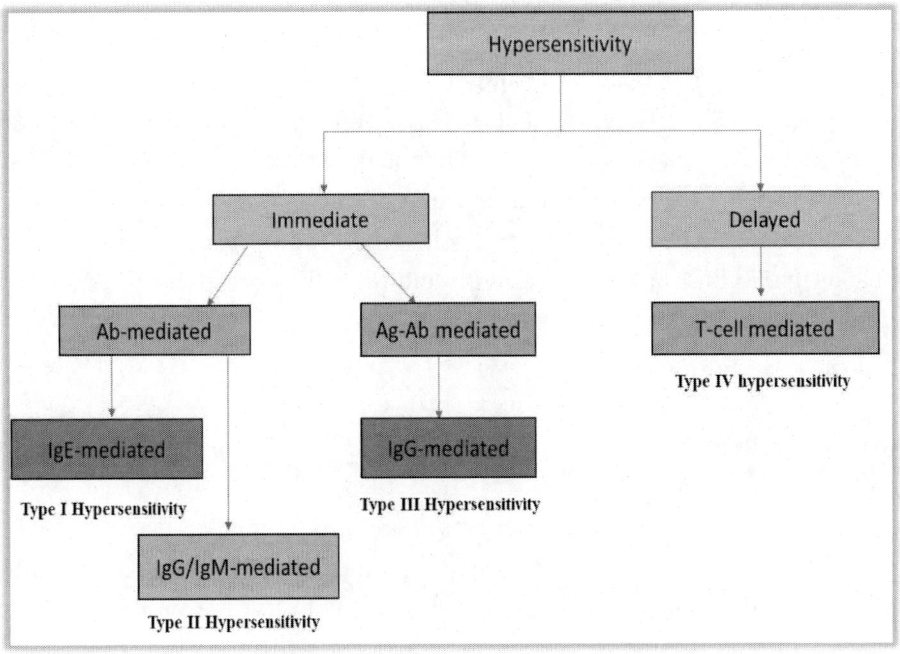

Figure 1.1. Represents the overview of hypersensitivity.

The same immune reactions that protect us from infection can also inflict a great deal of damage, not simply on a pathogen, but on our own cells and tissues. The immune uses multiple strategies to reduce damage to self by turning off responses when pathogen is cleared and avoiding reactions to self-antigens.

However, these checks and balances can break down, leading to immune-mediated reactions that are more detrimental than protective. Some immune-mediated disorders are caused by a failure of immune tolerance. Others are caused by an inappropriately vigorous innate and/or adaptive response to antigens that pose little or no threat. These disorders, called *hypersensitivities,* will be the main focus of this chapter. Finally, some disorders are caused by a failure to turn off innate or adaptive responses, resulting in a chronic inflammatory state.

Causes of Hypersensitive Reactions

Immune responses against antigens from different sources can be the underlying causes of hypersensitivity reactions. Substances that induce hypersensitivity differ widely in chemical nature. Some are frankly antigenic, such as foreign serum and egg albumin while others like plant pollens possess feeble antigenicity. Still others like drugs are completely non- antigenic but may combine with and alter the specificity of proteins. Some of the causes of hypersensitive are:

Autoimmunity

Autoimmunity is the response of the adaptive immune system to self-antigens that occurs when mechanisms of self- tolerance fail. Autoimmunity is one of the causes of hypersensitivity. It's pretty amazing that the immune system can produce ten million different cell types that each can respond to a foreign antigen, and it's even more amazing that, in most people, none of these randomly generated cell types reacts against self-antigens (Figure 1.2). Normally as the immune system is randomly generating some ten million different clones, it's constantly cutting the self-reactant ones from the final pool as they are created. If this process of getting rid of self-reacting lymphocytes fail or is incomplete, then B or T cells that may become activated against self- antigens will be produced. These rogue cells or their products can then react against self-antigens. This is the basis of autoimmune disease.

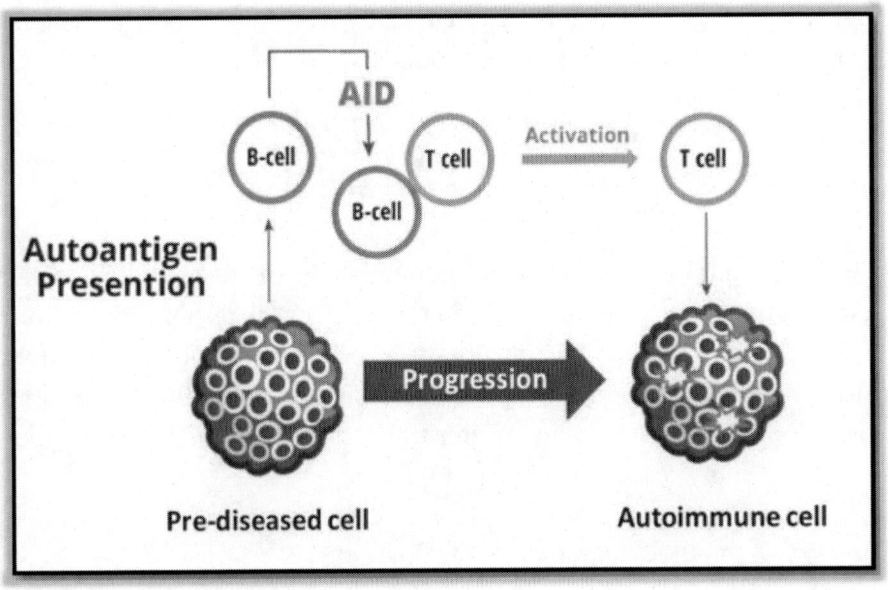

Figure 1.2. Represents the progression of autoimmune cell.

Reactions against Microbes

Immune responses against microbial antigens may cause diseases if the reactions are excessive or the microbes are unusually persistent. The antibodies are produced against microbial antigens to produce immune complexes that trigger inflammation in the tissues.

Reaction against Environmental Antigens

Most healthy individuals do not react against common, generally harmless environmental substances, but a significant percentage of population is abnormally responsive to one or more of these substances as a result of which such persons generate Immunoglobulin E antibodies that cause allergic reactions. In all these conditions, the mechanisms of tissue injury are the same as those that normally function to eliminate infectious pathogens. These mechanisms include innate immune responses, T lymphocytes, various other effector cells and mediators.

TYPES OF HYPERSENSITIVITY REACTIONS

Hypersensitivity reactions are commonly classified according to the type of immune response and the effector mechanism responsible for cell and tissue injury. This classification was originally developed by two British Immunologists, Phillip Gell and Robin Coombs- 1960. According to Gell-Coomb hypersensitivity designations, there are four different types of hypersensitivity reactions (Figure 1.3):

- Type I hypersensitivity
- Type II hypersensitivity
- Type III hypersensitivity
- Type IV hypersensitivity

Type I Hypersensitivity

Type I hypersensitivity is an allergic reaction provoked by re-exposure to a specific type of antigen which is referred to as an allergen. This reaction is also called immediate hypersensitivity because it begins rapidly, within minutes of antigen challenge (immediate) and has major pathologic consequences. Immediate hypersensitivity caused by Immunoglobulin E antibodies specific for environmental antigens and mast cells is the most prevalent type of hypersensitivity reactions.

Gell and Coomb's classification of hypersensitive reaction

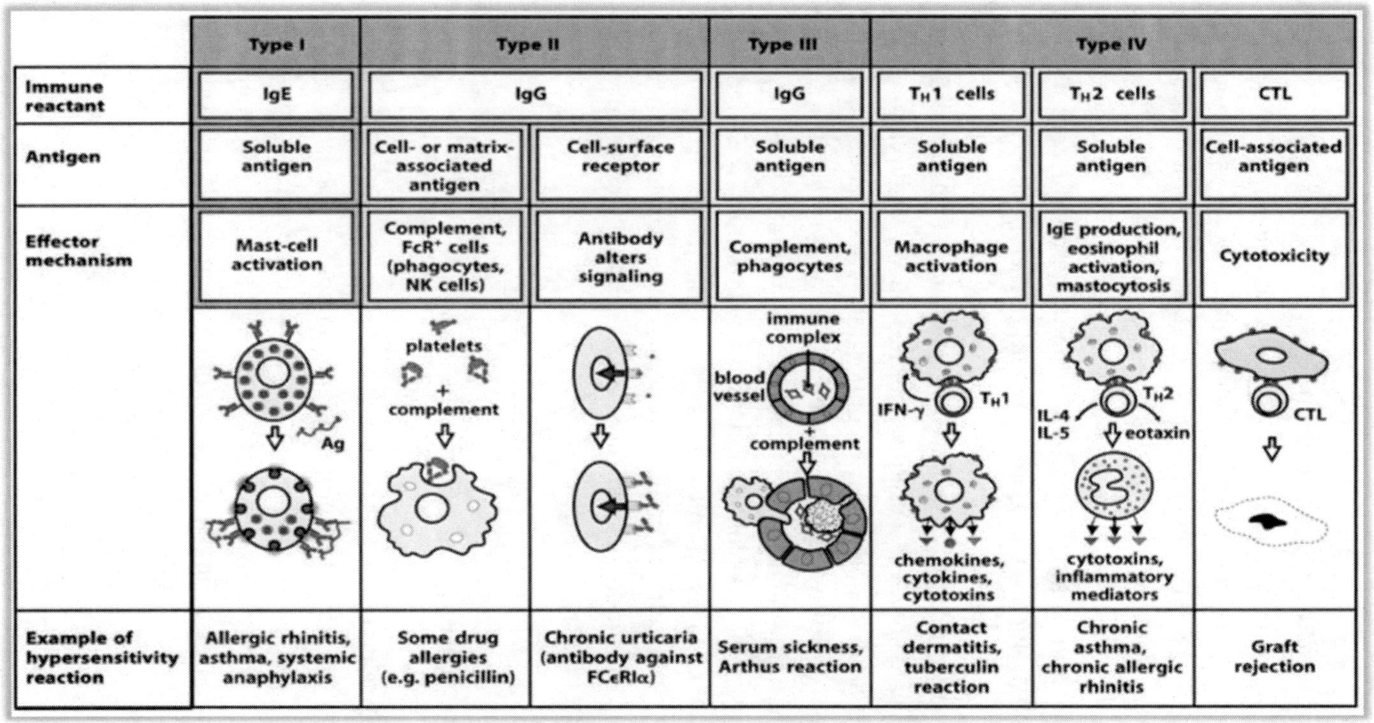

	Type I	Type II		Type III	Type IV		
Immune reactant	IgE	IgG		IgG	T_H1 cells	T_H2 cells	CTL
Antigen	Soluble antigen	Cell- or matrix-associated antigen	Cell-surface receptor	Soluble antigen	Soluble antigen	Soluble antigen	Cell-associated antigen
Effector mechanism	Mast-cell activation	Complement, FcR^+ cells (phagocytes, NK cells)	Antibody alters signaling	Complement, phagocytes	Macrophage activation	IgE production, eosinophil activation, mastocytosis	Cytotoxicity
Example of hypersensitivity reaction	Allergic rhinitis, asthma, systemic anaphylaxis	Some drug allergies (e.g. penicillin)	Chronic urticaria (antibody against FCεRIα)	Serum sickness, Arthus reaction	Contact dermatitis, tuberculin reaction	Chronic asthma, chronic allergic rhinitis	Graft rejection

Figure 1.3. Figure representing Gell and Coomb's classification of hypersensitive reaction.

Course of Hypersensitivity Type I Reactions

A variety of human diseases are carried by immune responses to non-microbial environmental antigens. These immune responses include the involvement of various immune cells such as TH2 cells, immunoglobulin E, mast cells and eosinophil. In these responses the antigens $CD4^{+}TH2$ cells, which then help B cells to produce Immunoglobulin E antibodies that are specific for the antigens and bind to the immunoglobulin E receptors on mast cells and blood basophils. When these cells associated immunoglobulin E antibodies are cross linked by antigen, the cells are activated to rapidly release a variety of mediators. These mediators collectively cause increased vascular permeability, vasodilation, and bronchial and visceral smooth muscle contraction. This reaction is called immediate response. Following the immediate response, there is a more slowly developing inflammatory component called the late- phase reaction characterized by the accumulation of neutrophils, eosinophils, macrophages and $CD4^{+}TH2$ cells. This later reaction is triggered by cytokines and by mast cells. In clinical medicine, these reactions are called allergy or atopy, and the associated diseases are called allergic, atopic or immediate hypersensitivity diseases.

Type II Hypersensitivity

Type II hypersensitivity is also known as tissue-specific or cytotoxic hypersensitivity. Type II hypersensitivity is a humoral response mediated by immunoglobulin G or immunoglobulin M that are produced against surface antigens on body cells. Immunoglobulin G and immunoglobulin M antibodies can cause tissue injury by activating the complement system, by recruiting inflammatory cells, and by interfering with normal cellular functions.

Course of Hypersensitivity Type II Reaction

Type II hypersensitivity is mediated by immunoglobulin G or immunoglobulin M targeting membrane- associated antigens. A sensitization phase leads to production of antibodies that recognize substances or metabolites that accumulate in cellular membrane structures. In the effector phase, target cells become coated with antibodies, a process termed as opsonization, which leads to cellular destruction by three mechanisms:

- Phagocytosis
- Complement dependent cytotoxicity (CDC)
- Antibody dependent cellular cytotoxicity (ADCC)

First the immunoglobulin G or immunoglobulin M antibodies coating target cells can bind to Fc receptors present on cells such as macrophages and neutrophils and mediate phagocytosis.

Immunoglobulin G or immunoglobulin M antibodies can also activate complement system via the classical pathway. Complement activation leads to the production of Membrane Attack Complexes, which forms pores in cellular membranes resulting in cytolysis (CDC).

A quite distinct cytotoxic mechanism, antibody dependent cellular cytotoxicity (ADCC) occurs when target cells coated with antibody are killed through an extra-cellular non-phagocytic process involving leukocytes that bind to the target by their specific Fc receptors.

Type III Hypersensitivity Reaction

This type of hypersensitivity is also called as Immune complex mediated hypersensitivity. This reaction is mediated by immune antigen antibody complexes which promote tissue damage primarily through complement activation. Hypersensitivity type III reactions involve the interaction of immunoglobulin G or immunoglobulin M with antigens to form immune complexes. It in turn triggers classical complement activation, leading to overproduction of other inflammatory mediators, leading to recruitment, activation and degranulation of peripheral blood granulocytes such as basophils or an influx of migrating neutrophils to specific tissues such as kidneys, lungs and joints culminating the damage.

Course of Hypersensitivity Type III Reaction

The formation of antigen antibody complexes occurs as a normal part on adaptive immune response. It is usually followed by Fc-receptor mediated recognition of the complexes by the phagocytes which engulf and destroy them and/or by complement activation resulting in the lysis of the cells on which the immune complexes are found. However, under certain conditions, immune complexes are inefficiently cleared and may be deposited in the blood vessels or tissues setting the stage for type III hypersensitivity response. These conditions include

- Presence of antigens capable of generating particularly extensive antigen – antibody lattices.
- A high intrinsic affinity of antigens for a particular tissue.
- The presence of highly charged antigens which can affect immune complex engulfment, and
- A compromised phagocytic system.

All these have been associated with the initiation of a type III response.

Immune complexes bind to mast cells, neutrophils and macrophages via the Fc receptors, triggering the release of vasoactive mediators and inflammatory cytokines, which interact with the capillary epithelium and increase the permeability of the blood vessel walls. Immune complexes then move through the capillary walls and into the tissues where they are deposited and set up a localized inflammatory response.

Complement fixation results in the production of anaphylatoxin, chemokines C3a and C5a which attract more neutrophils and macrophages. These in turn are further activated by immune complexes binding to their Fc receptors to secrete proinflammatory chemokines and cytokines, prostaglandins and proteases. Proteases digest the basement membrane proteins collagen, elastin and cartilage. Tissue damage is further mediated by oxygen free radicals released by the activated neutrophils. In addition, immune complex interacts with platelets and induce the formation of tiny clots.

Type IV Hypersensitivity Reaction

Type IV hypersensitivity reaction is commonly referred to as Delayed type hypersensitivity and it is the only hypersensitivity category that is purely cell-mediated, rather than antibody mediated. Delayed type hypersensitivity is an injurious cytokine-mediated inflammatory reaction resulting from the activation of T cells. The reaction is called hypersensitivity because It reflects excessive i.e., injurious immune responses and delayed because it typically develops during 24 to 48 hours after antigen challenge. Whereas antibody can be present in a preformed state, antigen-specific T cells need time to proliferate and then synthesize and secrete cytokines – hence referred to as “Delayed Type Hypersensitivity.”

Course of Hypersensitivity Type IV Reaction

Delayed type hypersensitivity (DTH) is a T cell mediated inflammatory response in which the stimulation of antigen specific effector T cell leads to macrophage activation and localized inflammation and edema within tissues. The T cell response may be directed against exogenous agents, such as microbial antigens and sensitizing chemicals or against self-antigens. After 4 hours after the injection of antigens, neutrophils accumulate around the post capillary venules at the injection site by about 12 hours, the injection site becomes infiltrated by T cells and blood monocytes, also organized in a perivenular distribution. The endothelial cells lining these venules become plump, show increased biosynthetic organelles and become leaky to plasma macromolecules. Helper T cells also assist cytotoxic T cell precursors to become killer T cells that can cause damage to virally infect target cells. Fibrinogen escapes from the blood vessels into the surrounding tissues, where it is converted into fibrin. The deposition of fibrin, and to a lesser extent, the accumulation of T cells and monocytes within the extravascular tissue space around the injection site cause the tissue to swell and become firm.

ALLERGY-CONCEPT AND DEFINITION

Allergy can be defined as an abnormal sensitivity to an ordinarily harmless substance, called "allergen" that produces a hypersensitivity reaction in response to the immune system's detections of the substance's presence. Today, we define allergy as immunological hypersensitivity that can lead to a variety of different diseases via different path mechanisms and thus different approaches in diagnosis, therapy and prevention can be taken. Allergies can be seen in almost every organ, most commonly in the skin and the mucous membranes." Allergology" is the science regarding allergic diseases and their differential diagnoses and mechanisms. It requires clinical experience in allergic diseases, basic understanding of the immune system in physiology and pathology and finally extensive knowledge of environmental factors in eliciting or modulating allergic reactions.

Allergy is not a disease itself, but a mechanism leading to disease. In clinical practice, allergy manifests in form of various different conditions such as anaphylaxis, urticaria, angioedema, allergic rhino conjunctivitis, allergic asthma, serum sickness, allergic vasculitis, hypersensitivity pneumonitis, atopic dermatitis (eczema), contact dermatitis and granulomatous reactions, as well as the colorful spectrum of food- or drug – induced hypersensitivity reactions (Figure 1.4). Allergies can be seen in almost every organ. Most commonly, however, it is the skin and the mucous membranes that are involved since they represent the frontier between the individual organism and its environment. Allergy often starts in the first three months of life but very rarely at birth, although there is a strong genetic background. Allergy in some cases does not persist over life-time; it starts and some patients may outgrow their allergic disease spontaneously. Many allergic diseases have a chronic course, but there are ways to cure. Allergic diseases can be influenced by psychological processes in a positive or in a negative way.

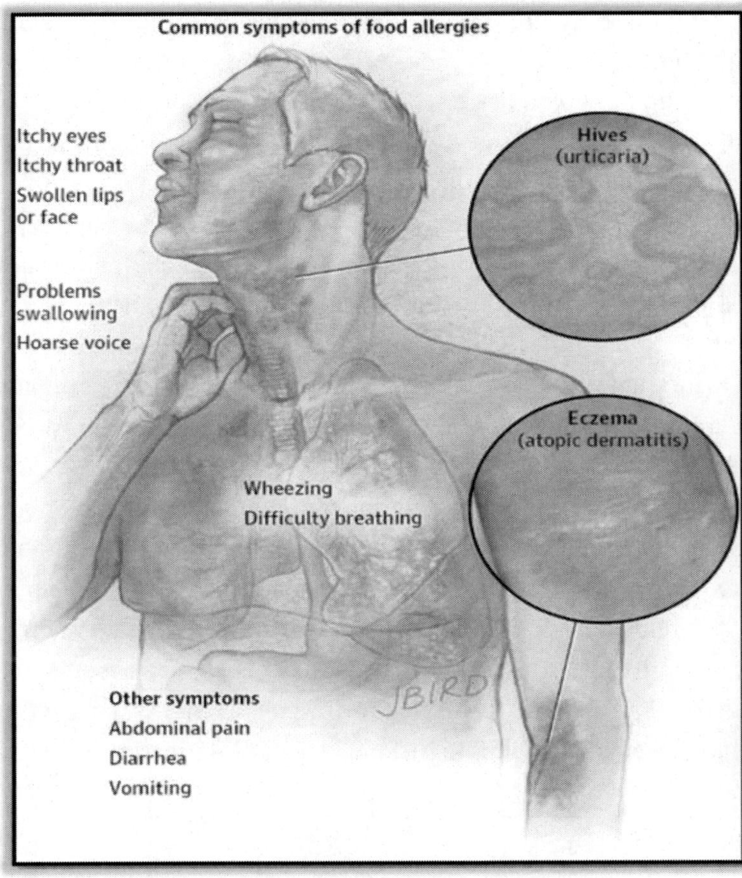

Figure 1.4. Represents some common symptoms of food allergies.

TYPES OF ALLERGY

An allergy starts when our immune system mistakes a normally harmless substance for a dangerous invader. This invader is known as "allergen" and the immune system then produces antibodies that remain on the alert for that particular allergen. Allergens are present both indoors as well as outdoors. The most common outdoor allergens are the pollens of grasses, trees or weeds, each with specific seasons. Characteristically, the higher the exposure to pollen, the higher the prevalence of immunoglobulin E antibodies, the higher the concentration of Immunoglobulin E antibodies; and the greater the severity of the seasonal symptoms. Pollen grains release species-specific proteins that act to trigger formation of a pollen tube. Exposure to outdoor allergens depends on the number of airborne particles, the time spent outdoors, and the efficiency with which the indoor environment is isolated from the outdoors. Any foreign species that exists indoors can contribute to the allergens found in a house dust extract. Most of the major sources of indoor allergens are well established i.e., dust mites, cat, dog, rodents, cockroach and a variety of molds. A wide range of environmental and lifestyle factors can contribute to "allergic" diseases. Furthermore, it is likely that these factors interact with each other in causing symptoms or exacerbations of disease. Chemical and particulate air pollution can play a major role in some regions of the world and there is good evidence that those effects are exaggerated amongst allergic patients. For air pollution, the effects appear to be directly related to dose, however in some studies the maximum effect appears to be 24 to 48 hours post maximum exposure. Depending on the type of allergen which has invaded the immune system of an organism, allergies have been classified into different types (Figure1.5).

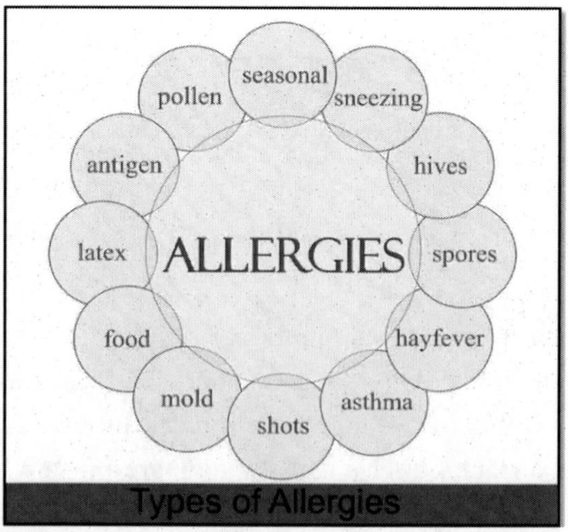

Figure 1.5. Showing different types of allergies.

Hay Fever-Allergic Rhinitis

Allergic rhinitis ("Hay fever") is the most common of the allergic diseases and refers to nasal symptoms that are due to aeroallergens. Year-round, or perennial, allergic rhinitis is usually caused by indoor allergens, such as dust mites, animal dander, or molds. Seasonal allergic rhinitis is typically caused by tree, grass, or weed pollens. Many individuals have a combination of both seasonal and perennial allergies. The cross-linking of allergens with allergen-specific Immunoglobulin E on the surface of mast cells leads to a rapid release of preformed mediators like histamine causing the symptoms of the early nasal response, i.e., sneezing, rhinorrhea and nasal itching. Symptoms result from the inflammation of the tissues that line the inside of the nose after exposure to allergens. The eyes, ears, sinuses, and throat can also be involved. The most common symptoms include the following:

- Runny_nose
- Stuffy nose
- Sneezing
- Itchy nose, eyes, ears, and throat
- Postnasal drip (throat clearing)

Asthma

Asthma is a respiratory condition that results from inflammation and hyper reactivity of the airways, leading to recurrent, reversible narrowing of the airways. Asthma can often coexist with allergic rhinitis. In the current update of the Global Initiative for Asthma, asthma is described as a heterogeneous disease, usually characterized by airway inflammation, and defined by the presence of respiratory symptoms such as wheeze, shortness of breath, chest tightness and cough that vary over time and in intensity, together with variable expiratory airflow limitation. It is a chronic respiratory disease that can affect 1 to 18% of the population with considerable variability among countries. Symptoms and airflow limitation may resolve spontaneously or in response to medication, and may sometimes be absent for weeks or months at a time. Patients can experience episodic flare-ups (exacerbations) of asthma that may be life-threatening and carry a significant burden to patients and the community. The variation of symptoms over time is triggered by factors such as exercise, allergen exposure, weather, or viral respiratory infections. Other common triggers include respiratory viral infections and exercise. Common symptoms include the following:

- Shortness of breath
- Wheezing
- Coughing
- Chest tightness

Conjunctivitis

Allergic eyes (conjunctivitis) are inflammation of the tissue layers (membranes) that covers the surface of the eyeball and the undersurface of the eyelid. Allergic conjunctivitis (AC) refers to a broad group of disorders involving inflammation of the conjunctiva and presents in a number of forms. It is the most common ocular allergic disorder affecting approximately 25% of the population and is responsible for presentation to a number of doctors including general practitioners, allergists and ophthalmologists. The characteristics of Allergic Conjunctivitis include ocular itch, tearing, redness, chemosis and lid edema. Itch is considered a hallmark symptom but may also be experienced in those with dry eye. Signs are usually more dramatic and obvious in those with Seasonal Allergic Conjunctivitis compared to those with Perennial Allergic Conjunctivitis. Seasonal and perennial Allergic Conjunctivitis (SAC and PAC) are the most common forms and most frequently occur with nasal allergy. They are caused by a classic type 1 hypersensitivity reaction to common aeroallergens Dry eye syndrome results from decreased tear production or disruption to the tear film stability. It can be confused with allergy and can commonly co-exist with Allergic Conjunctivitis. It is worsened by the use of oral antihistamines. The inflammation occurs as a result of an allergic reaction and may produce the following symptoms, which are generally present in both eyes (Figure 1.6):

- Redness under the lids and of the eye overall
- Watery, itchy eyes
- Swelling of the membranes

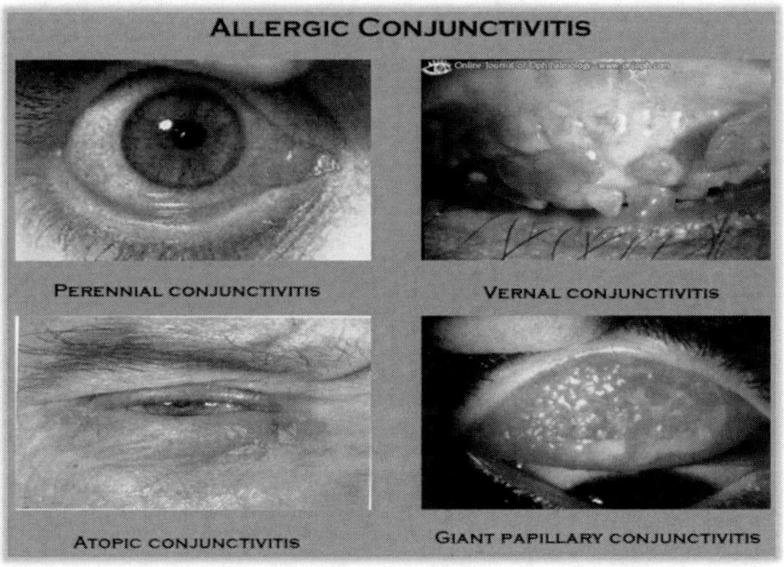

Figure 1.6. Represents different types of conjunctivitis.

Eczema (Atopic Dermatitis)

Eczema (Atopic Dermatitis) is a condition commonly found in infants. It tends to occur in individuals at risk for other allergic conditions (asthma and allergic rhinitis) but is not usually caused by direct allergen exposure.

Atopic Dermatitis (AD) is the most common chronic inflammatory skin disease and may represent the very initial phase of the so called atopic march. The incidence of Atopic Dermatitis has increased by two- to three-fold during the past three decades in industrialized countries. Atopic Dermatitis affects up to 20% of the children and 2 to 10% of adults and has a deep impact on the quality of life of patients and parents. The increasing prevalence may be linked to the Western lifestyle. Due to its complex pathophysiology, the natural history of Atopic Dermatitis is highly variable and may be determined by a number of (epi) genetic as well as environmental factors including the recently identified microbiome (Figure 1.7). About 30% of the children, who have started the disease in the first

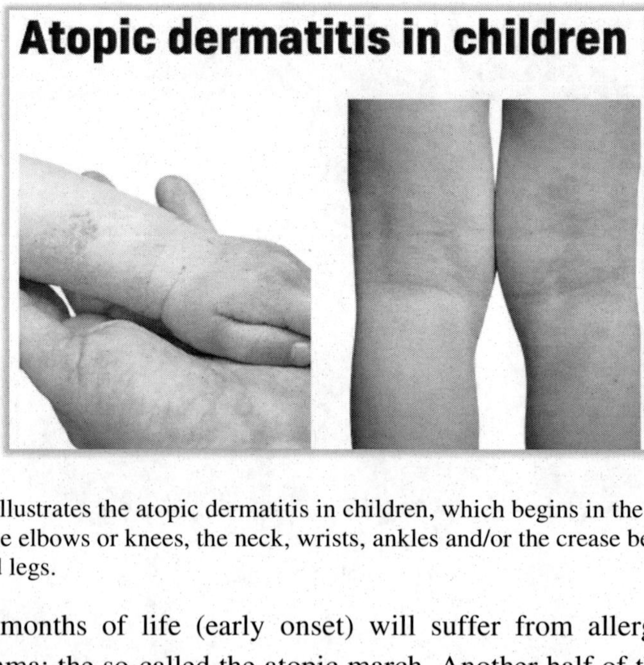

Figure 1.7. Illustrates the atopic dermatitis in children, which begins in the inside creases of the elbows or knees, the neck, wrists, ankles and/or the crease between the buttocks and legs.

weeks or months of life (early onset) will suffer from allergic rhinitis and/or asthma: the so-called the atopic march. Another half of the affected children will experience a remission before puberty. Social interactions, psychological adjustments, work success, sexual relationships, and quality of life often are dependent on the course of disease. The rash results from a complicated inflammatory process. Common features include the following:

- Dry skin associated with significant itching
- Involvement of the face, behind the elbows, and behind knees, though the rash can occur anywhere.

TREATMENT OF ALLERGIES

Allergy is a trigger for a variety of conditions. Allergy testing is directed towards establishing which triggers, if any, are responsible for the particular problems a patient experience. Once an allergic trigger has been identified, the management plan will depend on three main factors: (a) how easy it is to avoid the trigger, (b) whether there are multiple triggers and (c) how easy it is to induce tolerance.

The possibility of avoidance depends on the source for airborne allergens. Pollens and mold spores may be ubiquitous and so avoidance measures are impossible. In contrast, occupational allergens may be contained by alterations to manufacturing processes or air supply system. Animal dander's may be avoidable in one's own home, but may be a problem, if the patient has to visit other homes in the course of their work. Exposure to house dust mite allergens can be contained by exclusion covers, but has not always proved as effective as one might hope. In part, this may reflect the existence of multiple triggers, but it is also possible that the mechanisms, which lead to the induction of perennial allergic asthma and rhinitis, are not the same as those which lead to its perpetuation.

Drug treatment for allergies focuses on blockade of key mediators of inflammation (e.g., antihistamines and anti-leukotriene's) and more broadly on anti-inflammatory agents, principally glucocorticoids, which block the activation of key cytokines which augment and sustain airways inflammation. For full-blown anaphylaxis, self-administered adrenaline injection can be life-saving. More targeted therapies include monoclonal antibodies against Immunoglobulin E and against various pro-allergic cytokines (e.g., anti-IL-5). Although expensive, these therapies are useful in the management of selected patients. Tolerance implies that the individual either ceases to react or has a reduced reaction on exposure to allergens, which previously caused symptoms. Specific immunotherapy can do this by deviating the immune response away from the allergic pattern. The results are more impressive for anaphylaxis to insect venom than for airborne allergies, but there is no doubt some patients do extremely well. Recent reports of inducing tolerance in peanut allergy suggest that there is scope for further development of tolerance induction as a means of controlling food-related anaphylaxis.

CONCLUSION

Hypersensitivity reactions are a group of conditions in which the immune system, which normally serves a protective role, has a harmful effect. Both allergies and many autoimmune diseases fall under the umbrella of hypersensitivity, whereas autoimmune diseases involve a direct immune reaction to the tissues within the body. Hypersensitivity reactions are commonly classified into four types; Type I hypersensitivity reactions are immediate allergic reactions. Type II hypersensitivity reactions are referred to as cytotoxic, as they involve antibodies that are specific to particular tissues within the body and cause destruction of cells in these tissues. Type III hypersensitivity reactions are immune-complex mediated, with tissue damage caused by antigen-antibody complex deposition. Type IV hypersensitivity reactions are delayed and cell mediated, and is the only hypersensitivity reactions that involve sensitized T lymphocytes rather than antibodies. Substances that induce hypersensitivity differ widely in chemical nature. The original concept of allergy included all immune-mediated diseases and the term allergy was interchangeable with the term hypersensitivity: The term allergy was originally defined by Clemens Von Pirquet as “an altered capacity of the body to react to a foreign substance,” which was an extremely broad definition that included all immunological reactions. Allergy is now defined in a much more restricted manner as “disease following a response by the immune system to an otherwise innocuous antigen.” Allergy is one of a class of immune system responses that are termed hypersensitivity reactions. These are harmful immune responses that produce tissue injury and may cause serious disease. Almost every individual is allergic to some medium or the other in his/her lifetime. No human body is of the same composition and hence what could be allergic to someone can be harmless to another person.

MULTIPLE CHOICE QUESTIONS (MCQS)

1. Which hypersensitivity reactions are T cell mediated?

A. Type I
B. Type II
C. Type III
D. Type IV
E. None of these

2. Rheumatoid arthritis is an _______ disease that affects the _______

A. Allergic/cartilage
B. Autoimmune/nerves
C. Autoimmune/joints
D. Immunodeficiency/ muscles
E. Allergic/muscles

3. An example of a type III immune complex disease is

A. Contact dermatitis
B. Graft rejection
C. Serum sickness
D. Atopy
E. Allergies

4. Which of the following is considered an autoimmune disease?

A. Rheumatoid arthritis

B. AIDS

C. SCID

D. Agammaglobulinemia

5. A hypersensitivity reaction occurs

A. during the first exposure to an antigen

B. during a second or subsequent exposure to an antigen

C. in individuals with diseases of the immune system

D. Only in children

6. Arrange the following events in the proper order in which they occur during an allergic response.

1. Individual experiences symptoms
2. Individual is sensitized to antigen
3. IgE attaches to mast cells
4. Antigen binds to IgE

A. 1, 2, 3, 4

B. 1, 3, 4, 2

C. 2, 3, 1, 4

D. 2, 3, 4, 1

7. All of the following are associated with type I hypersensitivity except

A. Release of preformed mediators from mast cells

B. Activation of complement

C. Cell-bound antibody bridged by antigen

D. An inherited tendency to respond to allergens

8. To determine if a patient is allergic to rye grass, the best test to perform is

A. Total IgE testing
B. Skin prick test
C. DAT
D. Complement fixation

9. Atopic dermatitis is also often called

A. Acne
B. Eczema
C. Psoriasis
D. Hives

10. Antibody dependent cytotoxicity is associated with

A. Type I hypersensitivity
B. Type II hypersensitivity
C. Type III hypersensitivity
D. Type IV hypersensitivity

11. A positive blood test for allergy must include

A. Antibodies
B. Gluten
C. Antioxidants
D. Enzymes

12. An allergic reaction can produce urticaria. A common term for urticaria is

A. Atopic dermatitis
B. Eczema
C. Folliculitis
D. Hives

13. Allergies can best be described as

A. Sneezing, itching, watery eyes, scratchy throat

B. An overreaction from the immune system to a foreign substance

C. The onset of a cold during spring months

D. A reaction to the influenza virus during spring months

14. Which of these occupations is at risk for developing latex allergy:

A. Health care workers

B. Glove manufacturing workers, laboratory technicians

C. Estheticians, greenhouse workers

D. All of the above

15. The diagnosis of allergic contact dermatitis can be confirmed by

A. Tzanck preparation

B. KOH examination

C. Patch testing

D. Wood's lamp examination

ANSWER KEY

1.D, 2.C, 3.C, 4.A, 5.B, 6.D, 7.B, 8.B, 9.B, 10.B, 11.A, 12.D, 13.B, 14.D, 15.C

FREQUENTLY ASKED QUESTIONS (FAQS)

Q1. By derivation what does allergy mean and what does hypersensitivity mean? Are they synonymous?

Answer. The term hypersensitivity arose from the clinical definition of immunity as "sensitivity" which is based on the observation that an individual who has been exposed to an antigen exhibits a detectable reaction or is "sensitive" to subsequent encounters with that antigen. Allergy can be defined as an abnormal sensitivity to an ordinarily harmless substance, called "allergen" that produces a hypersensitivity reaction in response to the immune system's detections of the substance's presence. The term allergy is often used synonymously to hypersensitivity although it has a broader connotation and designates any altered activity, decreased as well as increased, to foreign substances. Both allergies and many autoimmune diseases fall under the umbrella of hypersensitivity.

Q2. Differentiate between antigen and allergen?

Answer. Antigen can be any substance (as an immunogen or a hapten) foreign to the body that evokes an immune response either alone or after forming a complex with a larger molecule (as a protein) and that is capable of binding with a product (as an antibody or T cell) of the immune response whereas an allergen is a usually harmless substance capable of triggering a response that starts in the immune system and results in an allergic reaction.

Q3. What are the most common symptoms associated with anaphylaxis?

Answer. Some of the most common symptoms associated with anaphylaxis are:

- Hives, present in 80%-90% of cases
- Nasal congestion, runny nose, itchy eyes
- Swelling of the tongue and/or throat
- Abdominal discomfort, nausea, vomiting, diarrhea
- Shortness of breath, wheezing, coughing
- Low blood pressure, leading to lightheadedness, passing out, or shock

Q4. What happens when you have an allergic reaction?

Answer. When a person who is allergic to a particular allergen comes into contact with it, an allergic reaction occurs. This begins when the allergen (for example, pollen) enters the body, triggering an antibody response. The antibodies attach themselves to special cells, called mast cells. When the pollen comes into contact with the antibodies, the mast cells respond by releasing certain substances, one of which is called histamine. When the release of histamine is due to an allergen, the resulting swelling and inflammation is extremely irritating and uncomfortable.

Q5. What are the most common causes of allergic reaction?

Answer. The most common causes of allergic reactions are:

- dust mites
- pollen (grass, weed or tree)
- foods such as peanuts, cow's milk, soy, seafood and eggs
- cats and other furry or hairy animals such as dogs, horses, rabbits and guinea pigs
- insect stings and tick bites
- molds
- medicines

Similar reactions can occur to some chemicals and food additives, however if they do not involve the immune system, they are known as "adverse reactions" rather than "allergy."

Q6. Which areas of body may be mostly affected by an allergic reaction?

Answer. Depending on the allergen and where it enters your body, you may experience different symptoms. For example, pollen, when breathed in through the nose, usually causes symptoms in the nose, eyes, sinuses and throat (allergic rhinitis). Allergy to foods usually causes stomach or bowel problems, and may cause hives (urticaria). Allergic reactions can also involve several parts of the body at the same time.

Q7. What are the effective treatment options available for treating an allergic reaction?

Answer. Allergen avoidance or minimization relies on identifying the cause of your allergy and then taking steps to reduce your exposure to the allergen. For instance, many people are allergic to dust mites. Therefore reducing dust mite in the house is important. Medications used to treat allergies include Antihistamines, Intranasal corticosteroid nasal sprays (INCS), Adrenaline and various combination therapies. Non-medicated treatments such as saline sprays are used for treating allergic rhinitis and sinusitis. Allergen immunotherapy (also known as desensitization) is a long-term treatment which changes the immune system's response to allergens. It involves the administration of regular, gradually increasing amounts of allergen extracts, by injections or by sublingual tablets, sprays or drops.

Q8. Outline the course of process of opsonization in hypersensitivity type II reaction?

Answer. The process of opsonization in hypersensitivity type II reaction occurs by three pathways viz,

- Phagocytosis: First the immunoglobulin G or immunoglobulin M antibodies coating target cells can bind to Fc receptors present on cells such as macrophages and neutrophils and mediate phagocytosis.
- Complement dependent cytotoxicity: Immunoglobulin G or immunoglobulin M antibodies can also activate complement system via the classical pathway. Complement activation leads to the production of Membrane Attack Complexes, which forms pores in cellular membranes resulting in cytolysis (CDC).
- Antibody dependent cellular cytotoxicity (ADCC): A quite distinct cytotoxic mechanism, antibody dependent cellular cytotoxicity (ADCC) occurs when target cells coated with antibody are killed through an extra-cellular non-phagocytic process involving leukocytes that bind to the target by their specific Fc receptors.

Q9. What are the most reliable allergy tests available?

Answer. Skin prick tests using extracts of allergens and blood RAST or allergen specific IgE tests are most reliable tests for allergic reactions, while as Patch tests are reliable tests for delayed allergic hypersensitivity to chemicals, food and metals.

Q10. What are the most common allergic diseases?

Answer. The most common allergic diseases are allergic rhinitis, asthma, allergic dermatitis, contact dermatitis, food allergy and urticaria.

Q11. What is a food allergy and what food causes allergic reaction?

Answer. A true food allergy involves the abnormal response of the body's immune mechanisms to specific foods or food ingredients. Foods that commonly cause allergy in infants and children are egg, fish, shellfish, milk, peanuts, soy and wheat. Foods that commonly cause allergy in adults are soy, fish, shellfish, peanuts and nuts. However, food allergy may develop to any food that is included in the diet, and may develop at any time of the life.

Q12. What is pollen allergy?

Answer. Pollen allergy is an allergic condition affecting the mucous membranes of the nose and the eyes etc., usually characterized by nasal discharge, nasal congestion, and itchy and watery eyes, itchy nose, inner ears and roof of the mouth, that are caused by a hypersensitivity to airborne pollen, such as the pollen of trees, grasses, and weeds.

Q13. Define immune complex mediated (type III) hypersensitivity?

Answer. This type of hypersensitivity is also called as Immune complex mediated hypersensitivity. This reaction is mediated by immune antigen antibody complexes which promote tissue damage primarily through complement activation. Hypersensitivity type III reactions involve the interaction of immunoglobulin G or immunoglobulin M with antigens to form immune complexes. It in turn triggers classical complement activation, leading to overproduction of other inflammatory mediators, leading to recruitment, activation and degranulation of peripheral blood granulocytes such as basophils or an influx of marginating neutrophils to specific tissues such as kidneys, lungs and joints culminating the damage.

Q14. Enumerate the various clinical testing methods for the diagnosis of allergic reactions?

Answer. The probability that a patient has a particular diagnosis can be determined using a combination of diagnostic tests. Some of the allergy tests widely used are:

- Skin prick test
- Patch testing
- Radioallergosorbent test (RAST)

Q15. What are the various diseases associated with the occupational allergy reaction?

Answer. The allergic diseases that may be contracted as a consequence of exposure to sensitizing agents in the workplace are rhinitis, conjunctivitis, asthma, eosinophilic bronchitis, hypersensitivity pneumonitis, allergic contact dermatitis, immunologic contact urticaria and occupational anaphylaxis.

ASSIGNMENTS

Q1. Briefly describe the course, clinical findings, and mode of treatment of immune-complex mediated hypersensitivity?

Q2. Explain the mechanism of pathophysiology of allergic immune response?

Q3. Discuss the various diagnostic tests involved in allergy diagnosis?

Q4. Discuss the various possible underlying causes of hypersensitivity reaction?

Q5. What do you understand by anaphylaxis?

References

Abbas, Abul K, Andrew H. Lichtman, and Shiv Pillai. *Cellular and Molecular Immunology*. Philadelphia: Saunders/Elsevier, 2010. Print.

Black, CA. (1999). "Delayed type hypersensitivity: Current theories with an historic perspective." *Dermatology Online Journal*. 5 (1): 7. PMID 10673450.

Bzowyckyj AS, Stahnke AM. Hypersensitivity reactions to human insulin analogs in insulin-naïve patients: a systematic review. *Ther Adv Endocrinol Metab*. 2018;9(2):53–65.

Chen CB, Abe R, Pan RY, et al. An Updated Review of the Molecular Mechanisms in Drug Hypersensitivity [published correction appears in *J Immunol Res*. 2019 Jan 31;2019:2489429]. *J Immunol Res*. 2018;2018:6431694.

Coico, R. and Sunshine, G. (2015). *Immunology: A Short Course*. 7th ed. Wiley-Blackwell.

Demoly P, Hillaire-Buys D. Classification and epidemiology of hypersensitivity drug reactions. *Immunology and Allergy Clinics*. 2004 Aug 1;24(3):345-56.

Descotes J, Choquet-Kastylevsky G. Gell and Coombs's classification: is it still valid?. *Toxicology*. 2001 Feb 2;158(1-2):43-9.

Gelincik A, Demir S, Şen F, et al. Interleukin-10 is increased in successful drug desensitization regardless of the hypersensitivity reaction type. *Asia Pac Allergy*. 2019;9(1):e9.

Gell PGH, Coombs RRA, eds. *Clinical Aspects of Immunology*. 1st ed. Oxford, England: Blackwell; 1963. Section IV, Chapter 1.

Hwang MJ, Do JY, Choi EW, et al. Immunoglobulin E-mediated hypersensitivity reaction after intraperitoneal administration of vancomycin. *Kidney Res Clin Pract*. 2015;34(1):57–59.

Janardhanan M, Amberkar VMB, Vidyasagar S, Kumari K M, Holla SN. Hypersensitivity Reaction Associated with Abacavir Therapy in an Indian HIV Patient - A Case Report. *J Clin Diagn Res*. 2014;8(9):HD01–HD2.

Kuby Immunology, Judith A Owen; Jenni Punt; Sharon A Stranford; Patricia P Jones; Janis Kuby, New York: W. H. Freeman, ©2013.

Kumar, Vinay; Abbas, Abul K, Aster, Jon C, eds. (2014). *"Hypersensitivity: Immunologicaly Mediated Tissue Injury."* Robbins & Cotran Pathologic Basis of Disease (9th ed.). Elsevier Health Sciences. pp. 200–11. ISBN 978-0-323-29635-9.

Mitchell, Richard Sheppard; Kumar, Vinay; Abbas, Abul K.; Fausto, Nelson (2007). "Table 5-1". *Robbins Basic Pathology* (8th ed.). Philadelphia: Saunders. ISBN 1-4160-2973-7.

Nahm DH. Personalized Immunomodulatory Therapy for Atopic Dermatitis: An Allergist's View. *Ann Dermatol*. 2015;27(4):355–363.

Pichler WJ. Drug hypersensitivity reactions: classification and relationship to T-cell activation. In: *Drug hypersensitivity* 2007 (pp. 168-189). Karger Publishers.

Rajan TV. The Gell–Coombs classification of hypersensitivity reactions: a re-interpretation. *Trends in Immunology*. 2003 Jul 1;24(7):376-9.

Rajan, TV. (2003). "The Gell–Coombs classification of hypersensitivity reactions: A re-interpretation." *Trends in Immunology*. 24 (7): 376–9.

Riedl MA, Casillas AM. Adverse drug reactions: types and treatment options. *American family physician*. 2003 Nov;68(9):1781-90.

Roitt's *Essential Immunology,* Peter J. Delves, Seamus J. Martin, Dennis R. Burton, Ivan M. Roitt. Thirteenth edition. Wiley-Blackwell.

Stone SF, Phillips EJ, Wiese MD, Heddle RJ, Brown SG. Immediate-type hypersensitivity drug reactions. *Br J Clin Pharmacol.* 2014;78(1):1–13.

Uzzaman A, Cho SH. Classification of hypersensitivity reactions. In *Allergy & Asthma Proceedings* 2012 May 2 (Vol. 33).

White KD, Chung WH, Hung SI, Mallal S, Phillips EJ. Evolving models of the immunopathogenesis of T cell-mediated drug allergy: The role of host, pathogens, and drug response. *J Allergy Clin* Immunol. 2015;136(2):219–235.

Websites

http://www.sciencedirect.com
https://www.ncbi.nlm.nih.gov/pubmed
http://missinglink.ucsf.edu/lm/immunology_module/prologue/
https://www.myvmc.com/diseases/hypersensitivity-reaction
https://www.amboss.com/us/knowledge/Hypersensitivity_reactions

In: The Fundamentals of Hypersensitivities … ISBN: 978-1-53617-012-2
Editor: Manzoor Ahmad Mir

Chapter 2

GELL AND COOMB'S CLASSIFICATION OF HYPERSENSITIVITY

Nissar Ahmad Wani, Manzoor Ahmad Mir*, Hina Qayoom, Umar Mehraj, Safura Nisar, Bashir A. Sheikh and Syed Suhail
Department of Bioresources, School of Biological Sciences, University of Kashmir, Srinagar J&K, India

ABSTRACT

Hypersensitivity can be defined as a state of increased reactivity to a foreign agent usually acquired by a prior exposure to the same or a chemically related substance.The term hypersensitivity evolved from the observations of Richet and Portier one hundred years ago, who described the catastrophic result of exposing a pre-sensitized animal to systemic antigen. The resulting outcome, termed anaphylaxis, became the prototype of immediate hypersensitivity responses. Coombs and Gell in 1963 proposed a classification scheme in which allergic hypersensitivity of the type described by Portier and Richet was termed type I, and broadened the definition of hypersensitivity to include: reactions that

* Corresponding Author's Email: drmanzoor@kashmiruniversity.ac.in.

resulted from antibody–antigen reactions, including cytotoxic reactions which they termed type II and immune complex reactions of the Arthus type, which were termed type III reactions, delayed-type hypersensitivity responses were given the classification type IV to describe reactions typified by cutaneous contact reactions upon exposure to certain agents such as nickel.

Keywords: hypersensitivity, anaphylaxis, cytotoxic hypersensitivity, Fc receptors, delayed hypersensitivity, Ig E mediated immune response, grave's disease

OBJECTIVES

- To discuss hypersensitivity and its causes
- To give an outline of Gell and Coomb's Classification
- To study the Detailed Gell and Coombs classification of hypersensitivity
- To discuss the modifications made to the previous classification.
- And last but not the least to talk about the relevance of this classification.

INTRODUCTION

Hypersensitivity or hypersensitivity reaction is basically an abnormal sensitivity to an allergen, drug, or other agent, where the body reacts with an exaggerated immune response. The term was first used to describe anaphylaxis. Richet, in his historic experiments attempted to immunize dogs against the toxin of the Portuguese man-of-war (*Physalia physalis*) (Figure 2.1). Some dogs which were injected with the toxin and survived were used for a second time. Unexpectedly the second injection rapidly caused vomiting, hemorrhage, asphyxia and death. It was reasoned that the first injection had sensitized the dogs to produce a state of hypersensitivity and the term 'anaphylaxis' was coined from the Greek roots, "ana" and "phylaxis," to mean the opposite of protection. Also called intolerance, Hypersensitivity reactions include both allergies and many autoimmune disorders, the difference being that allergies involve an immune reaction to common substances in the environment, whereas autoimmune diseases involve a direct immune reaction to tissues within the body.

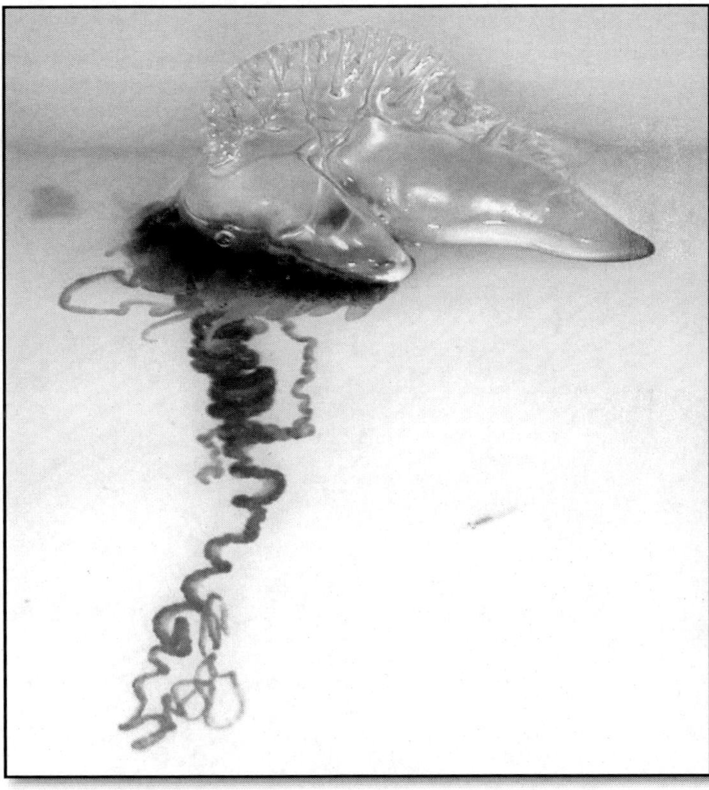

Figure 2.1. Represents the microscopic image of the Portuguese man of war.

EARLIER APPROACHES TO HYPERSENSITIVITY

The phenomena that constitute the basis of hypersensitivity reactions were discovered, and studies initiated, in the approximately 20-year period between Robert Koch's demonstration of a delayed hypersensitivity reaction to the tubercle bacillus in 1882 (Figure 2.2) and the demonstrations of anaphylactic, Arthus, and serum sickness reactions in the first decade of the twentieth century. Having discovered the tubercle bacillus, Koch showed that the delayed inflammatory response to an intradermal injection of the organism could indicate previous exposure to Mycobacterium tuberculosis in an asymptomatic person. This response became known as the tuberculin reaction and, as the Mantoux test, which is now recognized as the classical and best known example of a delayed hypersensitivity reaction Figure 2.3.

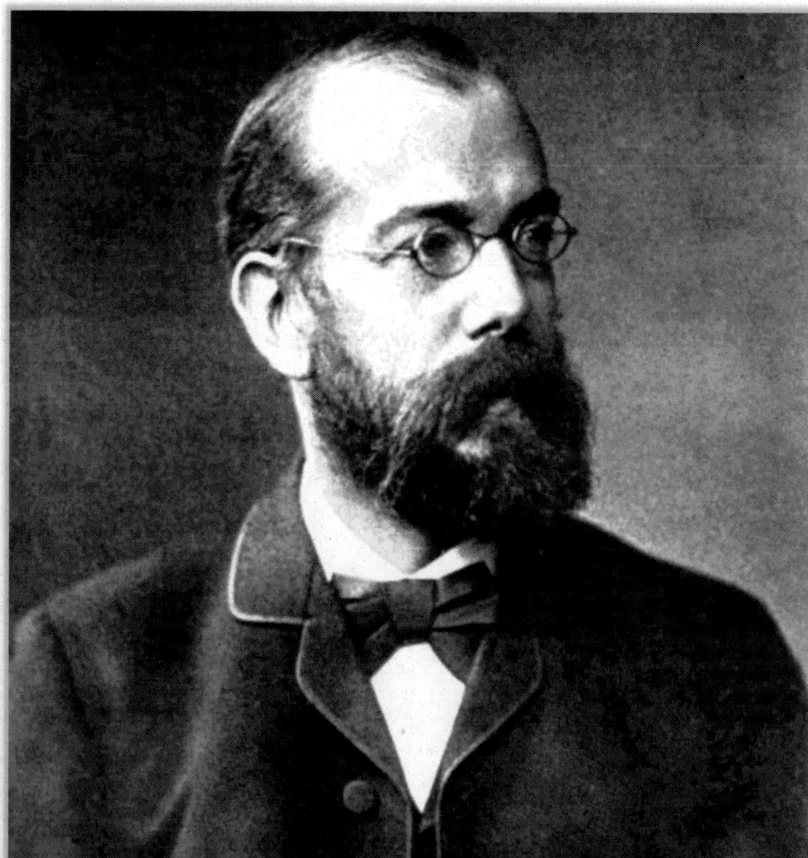

Figure 2.2. Image of Robert Koch, who originally described delayed type hypersensitivity.

Charles Richet by 1907 had shown that numerous proteins in small doses could provoke not "phylaxis" or protection, but "anti-protection" or what hc termed "anaphylaxis," and this state could be passively transferred to a normal animal by serum. In the first demonstration of the reaction which came to bear his name, N.M. Arthus in 1903 produced erythematous and edematous reactions in rabbits after repeated injections of horse serum, and in 1906, von Pirquet and Bėla Schick demonstrated the immune complex-mediated serum sickness reaction so named because it sometimes occurred following the administration of antisera prepared in horses. Despite Landsteiner's initial conviction that cell- bound antibody was the cause of contact sensitivity, Chase's experiments in 1941–1942 transferring "sticky," unclarified peritoneal exudate from guinea pigs sensitized by hapten–stromata conjugate with Freund's complete adjuvant led to the discovery that viable cells from the peritoneum, lymph nodes, and spleen-mediated contact sensitivity and tuberculin reactivity. 21 years after this Gell and Coombsproduced their classification of hypersensitivity reactions based on the immune mechanisms underlying the different reactions, that is, the latency of reactions, humoral or cellular involvement, complement involvement, and pathophysiological consequences for the host.

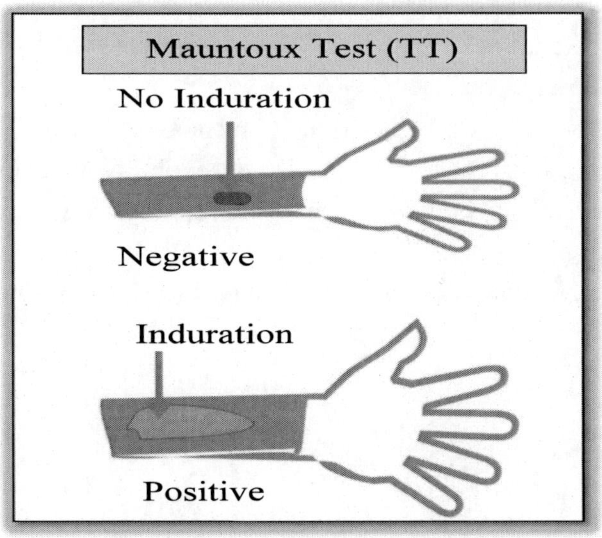

Figure 2.3. Represents the Mauntoux test (TT) for delayed type hypersensitivity.

Hypersensitivity Reactions Are Based on the Classification of Coombs and Gell

The adaptive immune response provides specific protection against infection with bacteria, viruses, parasites, and fungi. In particular, it is able to provide rapid protection against a repeated challenge with the same or a similar foreign organism or toxin. Some immune responses, however, give rise to an excessive or inappropriate reaction – this is usually referred to as hypersensitivity.

The term hypersensitivity evolved from the observations of Richet and Portier one hundred years ago, who described the catastrophic result of exposing a pre-sensitized animal to systemic antigen. The resulting outcome, termed anaphylaxis, became the prototype of immediate hypersensitivity responses.

Coombs and Gell in 1963 proposed a classification scheme in which allergic hypersensitivity of the type described by Portier and Richet was termed type I, and broadened the definition of hypersensitivity to include:

- reactions that resulted from antibody–antigen reactions, including cytotoxic reactions which they termed type II;
- immune complex reactions of the Arthus type, which were termed type III reactions;
- delayed-type hypersensitivity responses were given the classification type IV to describe reactions typified by cutaneous contact reactions upon exposure to certain agents such as nickel.

The original Coombs and Gell classification is shown in Figure 2.4.

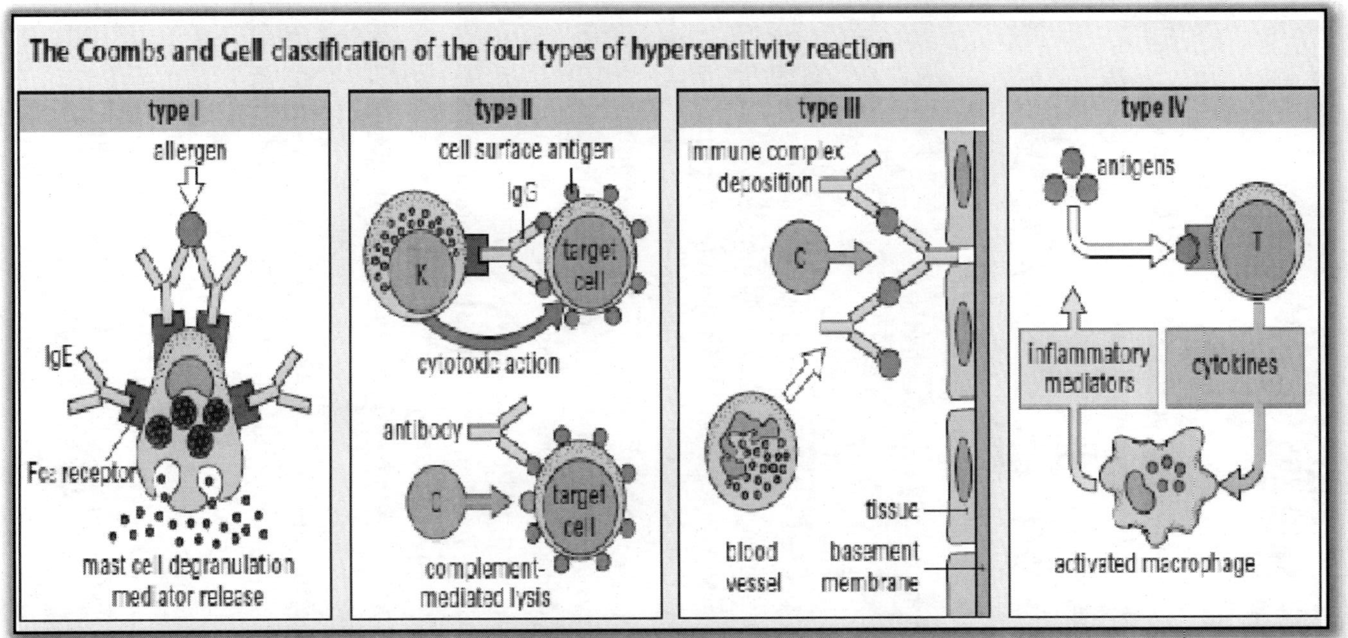

Figure 2.4. In type I, mast cells bind IgE via their Fc receptors. On encountering allergen the IgE becomes cross-linked, inducing degranulation and release of mediators that produce allergic reactions. In type II, antibody is directed against antigen on an individual's own cells (target cell) or foreign antigen, such as transfused red blood cells. This may lead to cytotoxic action by K cells, or complement-mediated lysis. In type III, immune complexes are deposited in the tissue. Complement is activated and polymorphs are attracted to the site of deposition, causing local tissue damage and inflammation. In type IV, antigen-sensitized T cells release lymphokines following a secondary contact with the same antigen. Cytokines induce inflammatory reactions and activate and attract macrophages, which release inflammatory mediators.

GELL AND COOMBS CLASSIFICATION

Philip George Houthem Gell was an immunologist working in postwar Britain. Together with Robin Coombs, he developed the Gell and Coombs classification of hypersensitivity (Figure 2.3). The Gell and Coombs's classification divides drug allergies into four pathophysiological types:

- Type-1 or anaphylactic hypersensitivity
- Type-II or cytotoxic hypersensitivity
- Type-III or immune complex hypersensitivity
- Type-IV or Delayed or Cell mediated hypersensitivity

The four types can be easily remembered by the pneumonic ACID which is A for Anaphylactic, C for Cytotoxic, I for Immune complex and D for Delayed. In the past several years it has become apparent that the Combs and Gell classification artificially divided mechanistically related antibody reactions (such as types I, II, and III), which contribute to the pathophysiology of many common immune-mediated diseases, while including the T cell-mediated reactions of delayed-type hypersensitivity (DTH) in a common classification (termed type IV). Based on our current understanding of the underlying pathways of inflammation triggered by antigen exposure and the disease conditions observed, common mechanisms appear to operate in types I, II, and III hypersensitivity (Table 2.1).

These common mechanisms involve the engagement by antibody–antigen complexes with cellular receptors for the Fc region of antibodies (termed Fc receptors). Understanding the mechanisms underlying these categories has resulted in the development of novel therapeutics based on the common pathways activated by these reactions and may result in the broader applicability of such therapeutics to multiple disease states.

Immediate Hypersensitivity Responses (Type I Hypersensitivity)

- have traditionally been referred to as type I hypersensitivity; and
- are characterized by the production of IgE antibodies against foreign proteins that are commonly present in the environment (e.g., pollens, animal danders, or house dust mites).

Antibody-Mediated Reactions (Type II Hypersensitivity)

- were previously referred to as type II;
- occur when IgG or IgM antibodies are produced against surface antigens on cells of the body.

These antibodies can trigger either by activating complement (e.g., autoimmune hemolytic anemia) or by facilitating the binding of natural killer cells (NK).

Immune Complex Mediated (Type III Hypersensitivity)

- involves the formation of immune complexes in the circulation that are not adequately cleared by macrophages or other cells of the reticuloendothelial system.

The formation of immune complexes requires significant quantities of antibody and antigen (typically microgram quantities of each). The classical diseases in which immune complexes are thought to be involved are systemic lupus erythematosus (SLE), chronic glomerulonephritis, and serum sickness.

Cell-Mediated Reactions

- were previously referred to as type IV;
- are those in which specific T cells are the primary effector cells.

Examples of T cells causing unwanted responses are:

- contact sensitivity (e.g., to nickel or plants such as poison ivy);
- graft rejection;
- the hypersensitivity skin responses of leprosy or tuberculosis;
- the exaggerated response to viral infections such as measles; and
- the persistent symptoms of allergic disease.

Table 2.1. Gell and coombs classification of immune-mediated allergic responses

Type	Mechanism	Manifestations
I	Ig E-dependent	Anaphylaxis,Urticaria
II	Complement-mediated cytotoxicity	Cytopenias
III	Immune-complex deposition	Vasculitis/nephritis
IV	Delayed-type hypersensitivity	Dermatitis or hepatitis

Table 2.2. Represents the types of hypersensitivity reactions

	Types of hypersensitivity reactions	
Types of hypersensitivity	Pathogenic immune response	Mechanism of tissue injury
Immediate hypersensitivity (Type I)	Ig E antibody, mast cells	Mast cell mediators
Antibody mediated (Type II)	Ig M and Ig G antibodies against cell and matrix antigens	▪ Phagocytosis ▪ Compliment ▪ Interference with cell functions
Immune complex mediated (Type III)	Complexes of circulating antigens and Ig M or Ig G antibodies	Compliment and Fc receptor mediated inflammation
T cell mediated (Type IV)	CD 4 and CD 8 T cells	▪ Cytokine-mediated inflammation ▪ Killing by CTLs

TYPE I HYPERSENSITIVITY

Type 1 hypersensitivity is also referred to as allergy. In the Gell–Coombs conception, disorders, such as hay fever or allergic asthma, are classic examples of Type I hypersensitivity. They implied that these disorders are driven predominantly by IgE bound to mast cells. On engagement of the cytophilic IgE with its appropriate antigen, mast cell degranulation and subsequent release of histamines, leukotrienes and other mediators that lead to inflammation at the site of allergy as blood flow to the affected tissues is increased (Figure 2.5).

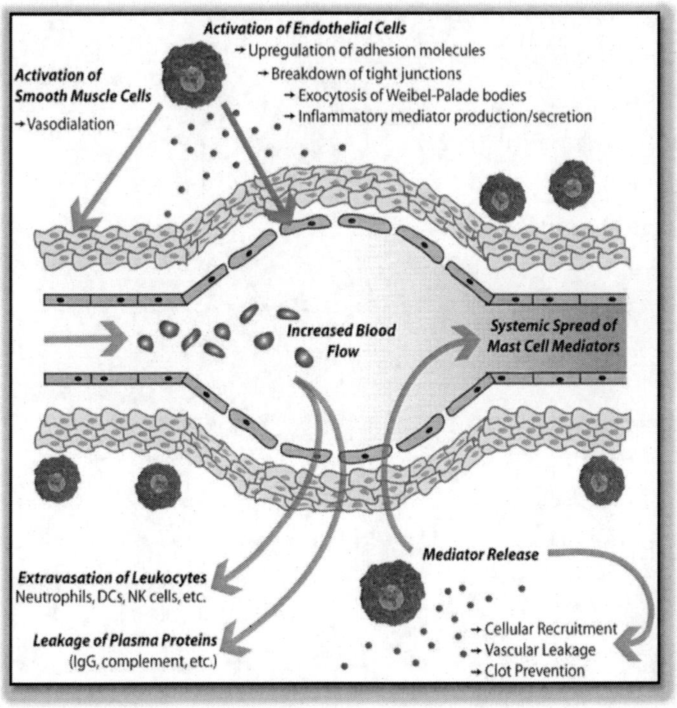

Figure 2.5. Illustrates the process driven by the allergic response mediated by type I hypersensitivity.

The allergic reaction in case of Type I hypersensitivity may be either local or systemic. Responses usually occur within 30–60 min but can be extremely quick (within minutes) and dramatic as in anaphylaxis. In some cases, a late onset reaction may also occur after about 3 or 4 hours of allergen exposure and the immediate reaction. Immediate reactions can affect a single organ such as the skin, eyes, bronchopulmonary tissue etc. causing symptoms ranging from minor itching and inflammation to sudden death.

A few examples of type I hypersensitivity includes:

- Allergic asthma
- Allergic conjunctivitis
- Allergic rhinitis ('hay fever')
- Anaphylaxis
- Angioedema
- Atopic dermatitis (eczema)
- Eosinophilia
- Urticaria (hives) (Figure 2.6)

IgE-mediated allergic reactions			
Syndrome	**Common allergens**	**Route of entry**	**Response**
Systemic anaphylaxis	Drugs Serum Venoms Peanuts	Intravenous (either directly or after rapid absorption)	Edema Increased vascular permeability Tracheal occlusion Circulatory collapse Death
Wheal and flare	Insect bites Allergy testing	Subcutaneous	Local increase in blood flow and vascular permeability
Allergic rhinitis (hay fever)	Pollens (ragweed, timothy, birch) Dust-mite feces	Inhaled	Edema of nasal mucosa Irritation of nasal mucosa
Bronchial asthma	Pollens Dust-mite feces	Inhaled	Bronchial constriction Increased mucus production Airway inflammation
Food allergy	Shellfish Milk Eggs Fish Wheat	Oral	Vomiting Diarrhea Pruritis (itching) Urticaria (hives) Anaphylaxis

Figure 2.6. Showing defined responses of type I hypersensitivity.

Sensitivity of an organism is normally assessed by their body's response to intradermal challenge with antigen. Some diagnostic methods used include:

- Skin prick tests
- Patch testing
- And In-vitro tests

TYPE II HYPERSENSITIVITY

Also known as cytotoxic reaction, this hypersensitivity reaction is characterized by antigen–antibody interactions, resulting in the local production of anaphylatoxin (C5a), the recruitment of polymorphonuclear leukocytes (PMNs) and the subsequent tissue injury due to the release of hydrolytic neutrophil enzymes after their autolysis. Type II hypersensitivity is mediated by immunoglobulin G or immunoglobulin M targeting membrane-associated antigens.

A sensitization phase leads to the production of antibodies that recognize substances or metabolites that accumulate in cellular membrane structures. In the effector phase, target cells become coated with antibodies, a process termed as opsonization, which leads to cellular destruction. The target antigens involved in type II reactions are often self-antigens. A number of different organs and tissues may be affected with the involvement of multiple underlying mechanisms. Reaction times can range from minutes to hours. Type II hypersensitivity reaction can occur in many parts of the body. Generally, they include Lungs, Blood system, Skin, Nerves, Thyroid etc.

The specific manifestations of Type II hypersensitivity are found to be:

- Transfusion reactions that occur due ABO incompatible blood transfusions.

- Drug induced reactions
- Rhesus incompatibility reaction due to incompatible Rhesus blood group transfusion
- Solid organ allografts
- And Autoimmune type II hypersensitivity reaction

Depending on the manifestations of different type II hypersensitivity diseases, there are different risk factors as well. There are some gender differences between diseases of type II hypersensitivity as well. Some diseases are more common in women such as Systemic lupus erythromatosus (SLE) (Figure 2.7) and Grave's disease. However, diseases such as Good pasture's syndrome are more common in men.

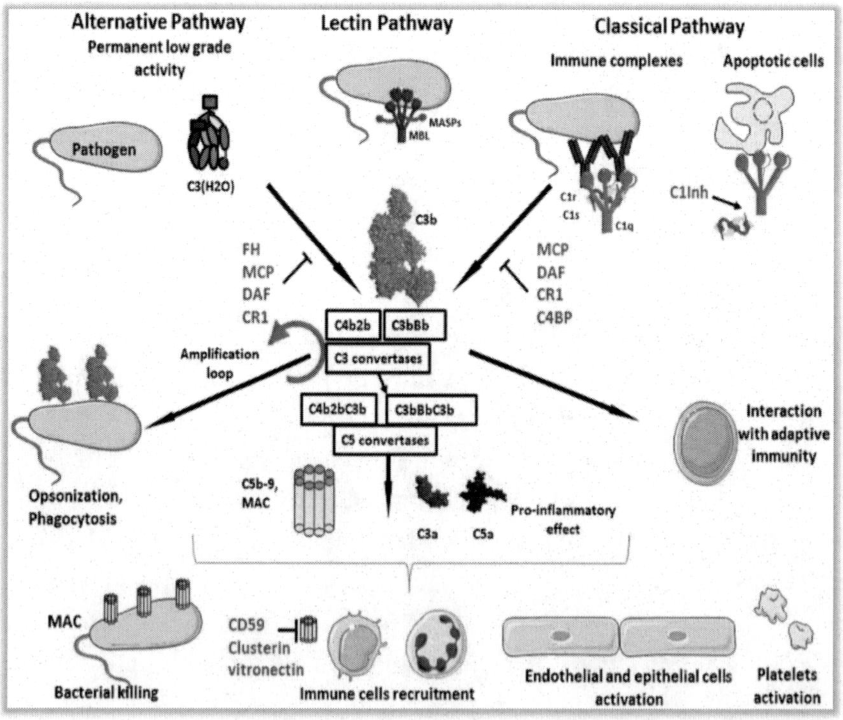

Figure 2.7. Illustrating the role of anaphylatoxins (C3a, C4a and C5a) in inducing type II hypersensitivity response. (Image Source https://doi.org/10.3389/fimmu.2015.00257).

TYPE III HYPERSENSITIVITY

In the Gell–Coombs system, type III hypersensitivity reactions also called immune complex hypersensitivity occur when antibody reactions occur in the blood, resulting in the formation of antigen–antibody complexes, which are deposited in the glomerular and/or pulmonary basement membranes. Deposition of immune complexes in tissues results in a tissue reaction initiated by complement activation that may lead to mast cell degranulation, leukocyte chemotaxis, and inflammation induced by the cell influx Figure 2.8.

After exposure, reactions may develop over a period of about 3–10 hours.The antigen–antibody complexes fix complement to release the anaphylatoxin products C3a and C5a. These induce the release of vasoactive amines from basophils, and chemotactic factors that attract platelets and other inflammatory cells, especially neutrophils. The reaction of antibody with antigen generates immune complex. In most of the cases, these immune complexes are removed from blood circulation. Some immune complexes are removed by phagocytic action of phagocytic cells in blood, others are first carried by blood to spleen where they are destroyed by macrophages.

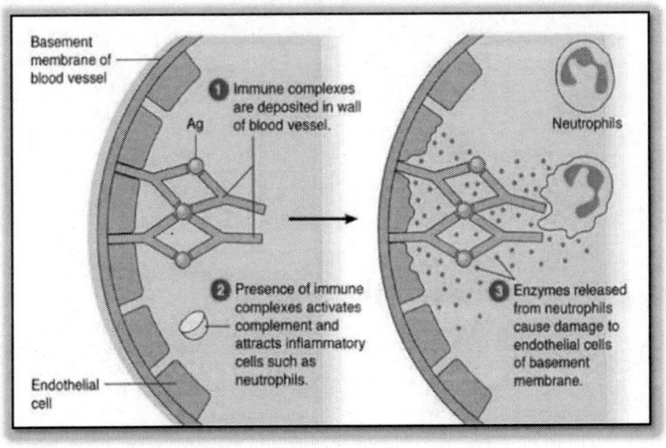

Figure 2.8. Illustrating the process of formation of immune complexes and its effects in type III reaction.

Complement system is also needed for removal of immune complexes from blood to spleen. In some cases, large amount of immune complexes is formed and deposited on various body parts and leads to tissue damage resulting in Type III hypersensitivity reaction.

If immune complexes are not removed from blood, they accumulate on wall of blood vessels and on tissue where filtration of blood and plasma occurs such as glomerular membrane, synovial membrane of joints etc. Type III hypersensitivity reaction is characterized by deposition of immune complexes on various tissues such as wall of blood vessels, glomerular basement membrane of kidney, synovial membrane of joints and choroid plexus of brain. Deposition of immune complexes initiates reaction resulting in damage of surrounding tissue and cause inflammation (Figure 2.9).

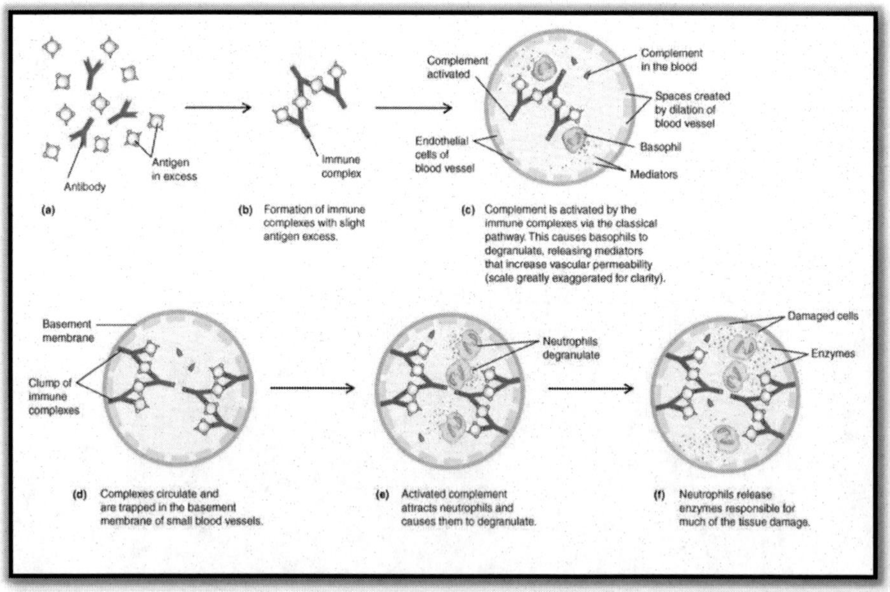

Figure 2.9. Diagram showing the overall procedure in induction of tissue damage.

Factors That Cause Deposition of Immune Complex and Increase Susceptibility to Type III Hypersensitivity Reaction

- **Persistent infection**
  In persistent infection such as Malaria, large number of immune complexes are formed and deposited in tissues.
- **Complement deficiency**
  Complement removes immune complexes from blood, but when complement system is deficient, large amount of immune complexes circulates in blood and deposits in tissues.
- **Autoimmunity**
  In autoimmune disease, large amount of immune complexes are formed and deposited in tissues.
- **Genetic defects**
  In certain genetic defects, small and soluble immune complexes are formed that cannot be phagocytosed

Detailed Mechanism of Type III Hypersensitivity Reaction

- Type III hypersensitivity reaction develops when immune complex activates C3a and C5a components of complement system (Figure 2.10).
- C3a and C5a are lymphotoxins (anaphylatoxins) that cause localized mast cell degranulation (Figure 2.9).
- Degranulation of mast cell releases histamine which increases vascular permeability of blood capillaries. This facilitates deposition of immune complexes on the wall of blood vessel.
- C5a, C3a and C5b67 also act as chemotactic factors for neutrophils, so they attract neutrophils at the site of immune complex deposition.

- C3b acts as opsonin by binding with immune complex. Neutrophils bind to C3b coated immune complex by means of type I complement receptor which is specific for C3b.

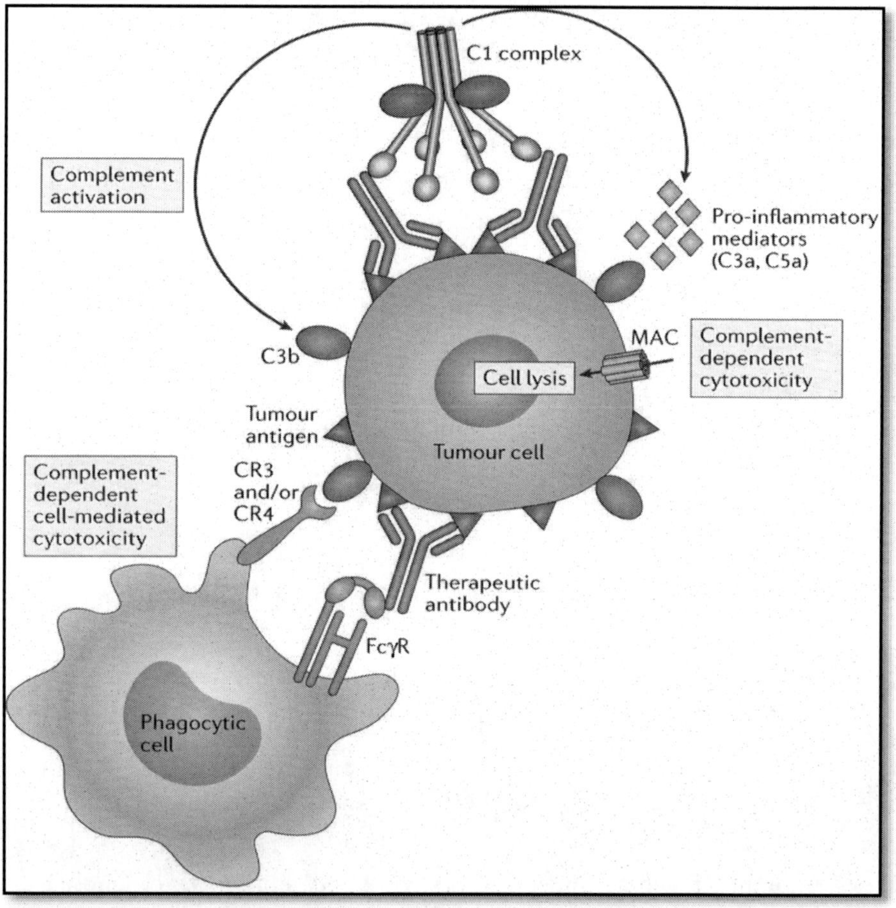

Figure 2.10. Illustrates the formation of immune complex and activation of phagocytic macrophage.

- The neutrophils attempt to phagocytose the immune complex but phagocytosis is not possible because immune complexes are deposited on basement membrane, so the neutrophil releases lytic enzymes to destroy immune complex.

- The lytic enzymes cause tissue damage in the surroundings of immune complex deposits, resulting in hypersensitivity reaction. Complement proteins can also contribute to tissue destruction.

Types of Type III Hypersensitivity Reaction

Localized Type III Hypersensitivity Reaction

- An example of localized Type III hypersensitivity reaction is Acute Arthus reaction.
- When an antigen is injected or enters intradermally or subcutaneously, it binds with an antibody to form a localized immune complex which mediates Acute Arthus reaction within 4 to 8 hours.
- As the reaction develops, localized tissue damage and vascular damage results in accumulation of fluids (edema) and RBCs (erythema) at the site of antigen entry (Figure 2.11)
- The severity of reaction can vary from mild swelling and redness to tissue necrosis.

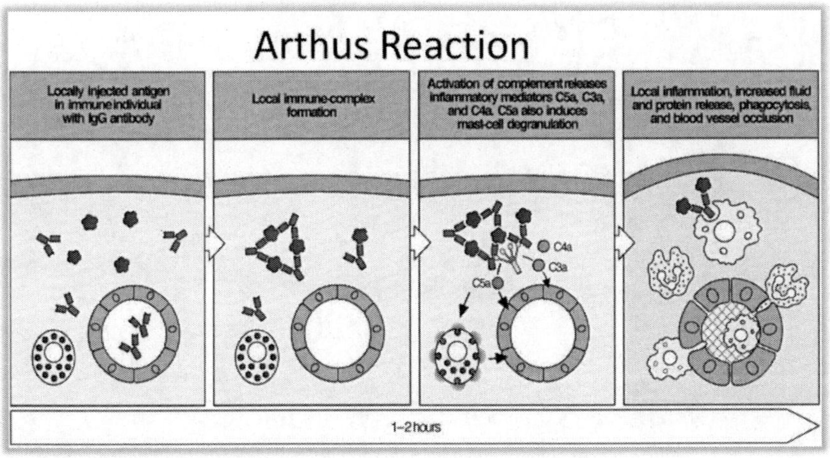

Figure 2.11. Represents the mechanism of Arthus reaction (Type III hypersensitivity).

Generalized Type III Hypersensitivity Reaction

- An example of generalized Type III hypersensitivity reaction is Serum sickness.
- When large amounts of antigen entersthe blood stream and binds to antibody, circulating immune complexes forms resulting in significantly excess antigens compared to antibodies, the immune complexes formed are smaller and soluble. Such complexes are not phagocytosed by phagocytic cells leading to Type III hypersensitivity reaction.
- The manifestation of serum sickness depends on the quantity of immune complex as well as the overall site of deposition. The site may vary but accumulation of complexes mostly occurs at the site of blood filtration.
- Generalized Type III hypersensitivity reaction at different sites results in different diseases such as Glomerulonephritis (acute Kidney inflammation) (Figure 2.12), vasculitis (inflammation of arteries), Arthritis (inflammation of synovial joints).

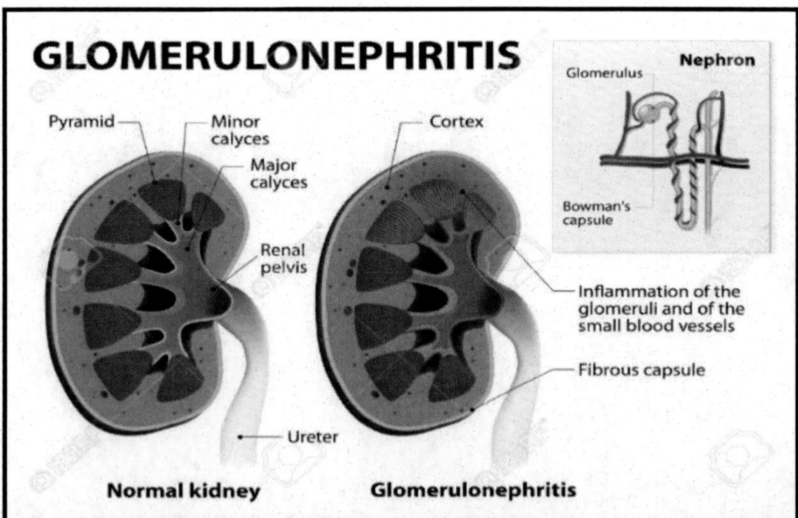

Figure 2.12. Representing the comparison between normal and diseased condition (glomerulonephritis).

TYPE IV HYPERSENSITIVITY REACTION

This type of Hypersensitivity reaction is also called as "Delayed type Hypersensitivity." Unlike types I, II, and III hypersensitivities that proceed with the involvement of antibodies, type IV hypersensitivity reactions are cell-mediated, in particular, by antigen-specific effector T cells. The term "delayed" refers to the cellular response that generally becomes apparent 48–72 hours after antigen exposure and distinguishes the response from type I or immediate reactions that often appear within minutes and peak in a matter of minutes or a few hours.

Type IV hypersensitivity is not represented by a single reaction. Rather, it is a number of related responses seen in a variety of reactions that may have beneficial or undesirable consequences for the host and which, at first sight, do not seem to have a lot in common except for their cellular immune base.

Gell and Coombs conceived several organ-specific autoimmune disorders as falling into the Type IV hypersensitivity reactions. One example would be insulitis, seen in the early phases of insulin-dependent diabetes mellitus. Here, the islets of Langerhans are infiltrated by a mixed cellular population comprising T cells, macrophages, natural killer(NK) cells and other leukocytes. Destruction of host cells ensues, by a combination of apoptotic death and cytotoxicity.

Type IV Hypersensitivity Reaction Occurs in Two Phases

The Sensitizing Phase and the Effector Phase

- Sensitizing phase
    - o Type IV hypersensitivity begins with the initial sensitization by primary contact with antigen. At first the antigen is processed and presented by antigen presenting cells (APCs) to CD4+T cell.CD4 +T cells are activated to form T helper cells (Figure 2.13)

- The T Helper cells are clonally expanded by binding with MHC-II molecule carrying antigen by appropriate APCs or antigen presenting cells. Varieties of APCs have been shown to be involved in activation of Delayed type hypersensitivity response including Langerhans cell and macrophages.
- CD4+ T cell are the primary cells activated during sensitizing phase of Type IV hypersensitivity response. However, in some cases CD8 + cells are also found to induce the delayed type hypersensitivity response.

- Effector phase
    - A subsequent or second time exposure to antigen induces the effector phase.
    - In this phase, TH1 cell secretes a variety of cytokines that recruits and activates macrophages and other non-specific inflammatory cells to the site of antigen injection.

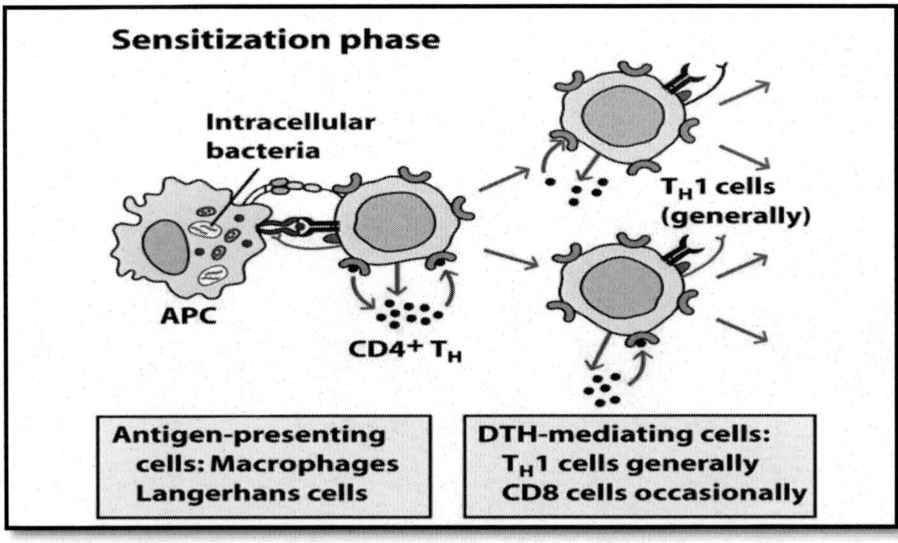

Figure 2.13. Showing the sensitization phase of Type IV hypersensitivity reaction.

- Macrophages are the principle effector of Delayed Type Hypersensitivity response. The activated macrophages exhibit increased level of phagocytosis and increased ability to kill the antigen (microorganisms) by various cytotoxic and lytic enzymes (Figure 2.14)

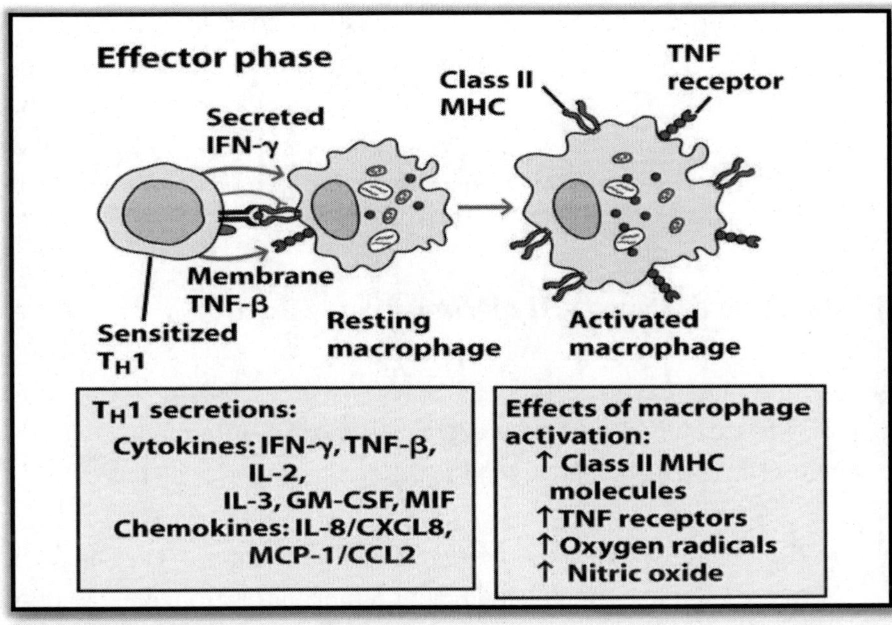

Figure 2.14. Showing the mechanism of effector phase of type IV hypersensitivity reaction.

- Activated macrophages releases lytic enzymes that damage surrounding tissues and intracellular bacteria.
- The influx and activation of macrophages in Delayed Type Hypersensitivity is important in host defense against intracellular bacteria and parasite, where circulating antibodies cannot reach them.
- Increased phagocytic activity and build up lytic enzyme from macrophages in the area of infection leads to non-specific destruction of tissues and intracellular pathogens.
- Generally, pathogens are killed rapidly with little tissue damage. However, in some case, especially if the antigen is not easily cleared, a pro-longed Delayed Type Hypersensitivity response can itself become destructive to host as intensive and

chronic inflammation develops into a visible granulomatous reaction.

- A granuloma develops when continuous activation of macrophages induces the epitheloid shape and sometime fusion of macrophages to form multinucleated giant cells. These giant cells displace normal cells forming palpable nodules and release high concentration of lytic enzymes which destroy surrounding tissues leading to necrosis.

Classification of Type IV Hypersensitivity Reaction

In some classifications, type IV reactions are subdivided into three categories based on the time of onset, the clinical manifestations, and the cells involved. The main features of the different categories includes:

- *Tuberculin type reaction (seen as local induration)* - The antigen is presented intradermally and reaction time varies from 48–72 hours. The main cells involved are lymphocytes, monocytes, and macrophages.
- *Contact type reaction (seen as eczema)* - This type of reaction occurs by cutaneous contact (e.g., with chemicals, poison ivy, nickel) and reaction time varies from 48–72 hours. The main cells involved are lymphocytes, macrophages.
- *Granulomatous type reaction (as in leprosy)* - In this case antigen persists in the host and the reaction time varies from 21–28 days. The main cells involved are macrophages, epithelioid, and giant cells.

Treatment of Hypersensitive Reactions

There is no cure for hypersensitivity. All the treatments aim at symptom control only. Depending on the severity of the allergic reaction, different treatment approaches are applied. Treatment options, either given alone or in combination, include the following:

- *Allergen Avoidance* - Prevention and avoidance of possible triggers are the mainstay of the treatment. However this is impractical in some diseases such as allergic contact dermatitis because some of the substance cannot be identified and remained unknown for a long period of time. However this is a useful and effective method for diseases with known external allergen. This method is not applicable for T-cell mediated autoimmune diseases such as type 1 diabetes mellitus.
- *Steroids* - These drugs are used for late phase of allergic reaction, and they include prednisolone, dexamethasone, etc. Depending on the diseases, steroid could become a long-term medication. In such cases, long term use will need medical supervision for monitoring of potential side effects.

  Other drugs that alter the body's immune system include interferon, cyclophosphamide, cyclosporine, etc. These drugs are used under specialist supervision.

ADDITION TO GELL AND COOMB'S CLASSIFICATION (TYPE V HYPERSENSITIVITY REACTION)

In addition to the four types according to Coombs and Gell, type V hypersensitivity has also been suggested. Type V is known as "granulomatous hypersensitivity, with differing kinetics from type IV and a specific macroscopic and microscopic morphology. Type V hyper-sensitivity reactions were additionally added to the scheme originally described by Coombs and Gell. Contrary to type IV and in agreement with types I, II, and III, respectively, they are mediated by antibodies too. The type V reactions are sometimes considered as a subtype of the type II hypersensitivity. As its mechanisms do not destroy target cells, they are responsible for induction of organ/tissue dysfunctions only most of authors prefer it to be and independent, the 5th type of hypersensitivity reactions.

Cells receive information from their microenvironment in which they live; they sense signals that process and transduce into the cell nucleus by means of second signals. The specificity of binding between the signal and its receptor is mediated by complementarities of structures. For instance, thyroid-stimulating hormone (TSH) released from the adenohypophysis, by binding to its receptors in membranes of the thyroid gland stimulates adenylate-cyclase system what results in production of hormones.

EXAMPLES OF TYPE V HYPERSENSITIVITY DISEASES

Graves' Disease

Morbus Graves is characterized by production of antibodies directed against the TSH binding receptor that subsequently stimulate the thyroid gland, resulting in production of hormones (thyroxine and triiodothyronine). Contrary to physiological situation, there is no feedback mechanism – the increased levels of the thyroid gland hormones do not stop its hormones production as at the physiological condition when elevated amounts of thyroxines switch off the production of TSH and subsequent synthesis of hormones. The result is the hormone overproduction and appearance of clinical symptoms of hyperthyroidism. As antibodies increase the function of a target organ, this type of hypersensitivity is also called stimulatory.

Autoantibodies not only stimulate cells of a target organ/tissue, they can also to inhibit it (hence the designation - inhibitory hypersensitivity reactions). A prototype of such a situation is *myastenia gravis.* It is an autoimmune disease characterised by production of autoantibodies directed against the acetylcholine receptors (AchR) present in neuro-muscular plates.

By occupying the receptors, they inhibit a physiological binding of acetylcholine to, resulting in precluding signal transmission and muscle activation. The result of the events is a paralysis of striated muscles. In some cases the anti-acetylcholine receptors antibodies activate the complement system; a destruction of cell present in neuro-muscular plates follows; the condition is more severe than in the previous situation and is incurable.

Pernicious Anemia (PA)

Pernicious anemia is a disease characterized by vitamin B12 deficiency caused by the absence of intrinsic factor. Vitamin B12 cannot be produced by the human body and must be obtained from the diet. When foods containing B12 are eaten, the vitamin is usually bound to protein and is released by stomach acid (Figure 2.15). Following its release, most B12 is absorbed by the body in the ileum after binding to a protein known as *intrinsic factor.* It is produced by parietal cells of the gastric mucosa and the intrinsic factor-B12 complex is absorbed by receptors on the ileum epithelial cells.

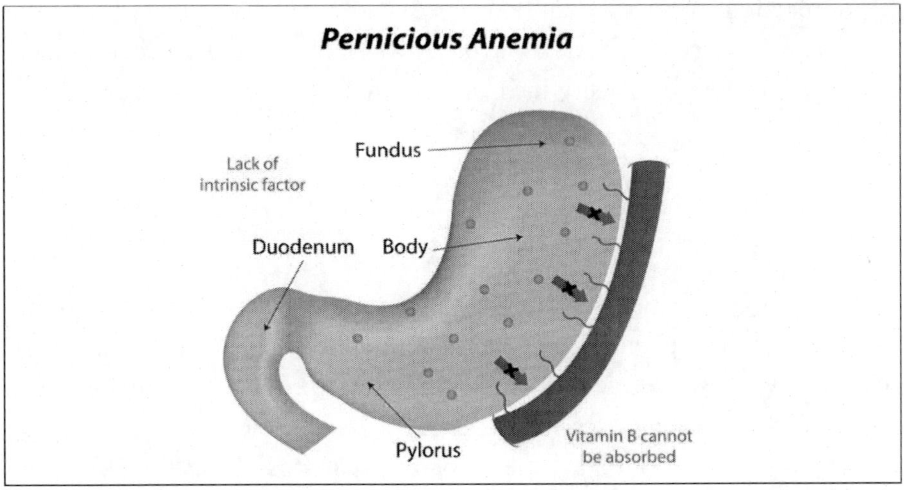

Figure 2.15. Representing the inability of ileum to absorb vitamin B12 because of the deficiency of intrinsic factor.

In patients suffering from PA, antibodies to parietal cells cause the destruction of the gastric mucosa, in which the parietal cells are located, leading to the subsequent loss of intrinsic factor synthesis. In other subgroup of PA patients, antibodies to intrinsic factor are directly induced. Without intrinsic factor, the ileum can no longer absorb the B12 and the disease develops.

How Relevant the Gell and Coomb's Classification Is Today?

Although Gell and Coombs classification was proposed more than 30 years ago, it is still widely used. But since only a limited number of drug allergies fit into this classification which do not include our current understanding of the immune response, its use is not recommended, particularly in the context of the preclinical safety evaluation of new therapeutic agents.

In fact, three different situations can be identified, namely pseudo-allergic reactions, primarily antibody-mediated reactions and cell-mediated reactions, which could serve as a basis for modern and more adequate classifications of hypersensitivities.

Conclusion

Immunological hypersensitivities are immune responses that lead to tissue damage. The phenomena that constitute the basis of hypersensitivity reactions were discovered, and studies initiated, in the approximately 20-year period between Robert Koch's demonstration of a delayed hypersensitivity reaction to the tubercle bacillus in 1882 and the demonstrations of anaphylactic, Arthus, and serum sickness reactions in the first decade of the twentieth century. The term was first used to describe anaphylaxis.

The Gell and Coombs's classification divides drug allergies into four pathophysiological types, namely anaphylaxis (type I), antibody-mediated cytotoxic reactions (type II), immune complex-mediated reactions (type III), and delayed type hypersensitivity (type IV). Although this classification was proposed more than 30 years ago, it is still widely used. Type I or Immediate hypersensitivity can range from acute episodic reactions to chronic debilitating disease, and is generally recognized to be increasing in prevalence within the "developed world" over the past 30 years. Type II hypersensitivity reactions represent damage resulting when the humoral immune system becomes directed against self. The mechanisms of type II hypersensitivity are those of antibody effector function. Type III or immune complex hypersensitivity results from the interaction of antibodies with antigen to form complexes. An example of type III hypersensitivity is serum sickness. Type IV or Delayed-type hypersensitivity reaction represents a T-cell mediated immune response and may be orchestrated by $CD4^+$ or $CD8^+$ T cells, depending on the nature of the target antigen.

MULTIPLE CHOICE QUESTIONS (MCQS)

1. Which of the following hypersensitivities are immune complex mediated?

A. Type I hypersensitivity
B. Type II hypersensitivity
C. Type III hypersensitivity
D. Type IV hypersensitivity

2. Which of the following are examples of type III hypersensitivity?

A. Multiple Sclerosis and Contact Dermatitis
B. Rheumatoid Arthritis and Arthus reaction
C. Allergies and Asthma
D. Myasthenia Gravis and Graves' Disease

3. Type IV hypersensitivity is mediated by?

A. T cells
B. Eosinophils
C. Erythrocytes
D. Neutrophils

4. The principal antibodies involved in type II hypersensitivity are

A. IgD and IgB
B. IgG and IgM
C. IgG and IgE
D. IgA and IgD

5. A condition in which individual fails to recognize its own parts as self and develops an immune response against its own cells and tissues is called

A. Phagocytosis
B. Inflammation
C. Necrosis
D. Autoimmunity

6. Graves' disease is an example of ____ hypersensitivity

A. Type I hypersensitivity
B. Type II hypersensitivity
C. Type III hypersensitivity
D. Type IV hypersensitivity

7. Which of the following does not involve cell-mediated immunity?

A. contact sensitivity to lipstick
B. rejection of a liver graft
C. serum sickness
D. tuberculin reaction

8. A positive delayed-type hypersensitivity skin reaction involves the interaction of

A. Antigen, complement, and cytokines.
B. Antigen, antigen-sensitive lymphocytes, and macrophages.
C. Antigen —antibody complexes, complement, and neutrophils.
D. IgE antibody, antigen, and mast cells.

9. Classification of hypersensitivity was given by

A. Robert Koch
B. P. Portier
C. Gell and Coomb
D. von Pirquet and Bėla Schick

10. Which of the following type of hypersensitivity is also called "immediate hypersensitivity"?

A. Type I hypersensitivity
B. Type II hypersensitivity
C. Type III hypersensitivity
D. Type IV hypersensitivity

11. A hypersensitivity reaction occurs

A. during the first exposure to an antigen
B. during a second or subsequent exposure to an antigen
C. in individuals with diseases of the immune system
D. Only in children

12. Type V hypersensitivity is also called as

A. Cytotoxic hypersensitivity
B. Cell mediated hypersensitivity
C. Stimulatory hypersensitivity
D. Delayed hypersensitivity

13. Delayed type hypersensitivity response occurs in

A. 3 phases
B. 2 phases
C. Single phase
D. None of the above

14. A transfusion reaction (ABO incompatible blood) is found to be specific manifestation of

A. Type I hypersensitivity
B. Type II hypersensitivity
C. Type III hypersensitivity
D. Type IV hypersensitivity

15. Which of the following is considered an autoimmune disease?

A. rheumatoid arthritis
B. AIDS
C. SCID
D. Agammaglobulinemia

ANSWER KEY:

1.C, 2.B, 3.A, 4.B, 5.D, 6.B, 7.C, 8.B, 9.C, 10.A, 11.B, 12.C, 13.B, 14.B, 15.A

Frequently Asked Questions (FAQs)

Q1. What does hypersensitivity mean?

Answer. The term hypersensitivity arose from the clinical definition of immunity as "sensitivity" which is based on the observation that an individual who has been exposed to an antigen exhibits a detectable reaction or is "sensitive" to subsequent encounters with that antigen.

Q2. List the Gell and Coomb's classification for hypersensitivity reactions?

Answer. In the early 1970s, P.G.H. Gell and R.A. Coombs proposed following method of classification of hypersensitivity.

1) Type-1 or anaphylactic hypersensitivity
2) Type-II or cytotoxic hypersensitivity
3) Type-III or immune complex hypersensitivity
4) Type-IV or Delayed or Cell mediated hypersensitivity

Q3. Give examples of each type of hypersensitivity reaction responses?

Answer. The example of type I hypersensitivity reaction is – allergic rhinitis.

The example of type II hypersensitivity reaction is – transfusion reactions.

The example of type III hypersensitivity reaction is – serum sickness.

The example of type IV hypersensitivity reaction is – leprosy

Q4. What immune cells are involved in immediate hypersensitivity reaction?

Answer. In Type I hypersensitivity response, plasma cells secrete IgE antibodies that bind to mast cells and basophils that then release histamines, a vasodilator, and heparin, a blood thinner.

Q5. Outline the two types of hypersensitivity type II reaction?

Answer. The two types of hypersensitivity type III reaction are:

- Localized Type III hypersensitivity reaction (Arthus reaction): When antigen is injected or enters intradermally or subcutaneously, they bind with antibody to form localized immune complexes which mediate acute Arthus reaction within 4 to 8 hours.
- Generalized Type III hypersensitivity reaction: When large amount of antigen enters blood stream and bind to antibody, circulating

immune complexes forms. If antigens are in significantly excess compared to antibody, the immune complexes formed are smaller and soluble which are not phagocytosed by phagocytic cells leading to Type III hypersensitivity reaction.

Q6. Define cytotoxic hypersensitivity?

Answer. Type II hypersensitivity is also known as tissue-specific or cytotoxic hypersensitivity. Type II hypersensitivity is a humoral response mediated by immunoglobulin G or immunoglobulin M that are produced against surface antigens on body cells.

Q7. Outline the classification of type IV hypersensitivity reaction?

Answer. Type IV reactions are subdivided into three categories based on the time of onset, the clinical manifestations, and the cells involved. The main features of the different categories in one such classification include:

- Tuberculin type reaction (seen as local induration): The antigen is presented intradermally and reaction time varies from 48–72 hours. The main cells involved are lymphocytes, monocytes, and macrophages.
- Contact type reaction (seen as eczema): This type of reaction occurs by cutaneous contact (e.g., with chemicals, poison ivy, nickel) and reaction time varies from 48–72 hours. The main cells involved are lymphocytes, macrophages.
- Granulomatous type reaction (as in leprosy): In this case antigen persists in the host and the reaction time varies from 21–28 days. The main cells involved are macrophages, epitheloid, and giant cells.

Q8. What types of tests are available for diagnosis of allergy?

Answer. Sensitivity is normally assessed by the response to intradermal challenge with antigen. Some diagnostic methods used are:

- Skin prick tests
- Patch testing
- In-vitro tests

Q9. What are the most common allergic diseases?

Answer. The most common allergic diseases are allergic rhinitis, asthma, allergic dermatitis, contact dermatitis, food allergy and urticaria.

Q10. What class of antibody is responsible for immediate hypersensitivity?

Answer. Immunoglobulin E is responsible for immediate hypersensitivity.

Q11. Discuss the difference between normal immune response to antigen in immunity and in type I hypersensitivity?

Answer. The difference between a normal immune response and a type I hypersensitivity response is that plasma cells secrete IgE antibodies that bind to mast cells and basophils that then release histamines, a vasodilator, and heparin, a blood thinner. This cause inflammation at the site as blood flow to the affected tissues is increased. The reaction may be either local or systemic. Responses usually occur within 30–60 min but can be extremely quick (within minutes) and dramatic as in anaphylaxis.

Q12. Compare the initiation response time of each type of hypersensitivity?

Answer. Type I hypersensitivity – 2-30 minutes

Type II hypersensitivity – 5-8 hours

Type III hypersensitivity – 2-8 hours

Type IV hypersensitivity – 24-72 hours

Q13. What do you understand by stimulatory hypersensitivity response?

Answer. Although Gell and Coombs only categorized only four types of hypersensitivity responses, a fifth type is sometimes added called as stimulatory hypersensitivity. In this response the antibodies do not mediate their effect via cytotoxicity but rather are directed to a cell surface receptor and act as an agonist leading to stimulation of cell. Hence also called as stimulatory hypersensitivity.

Q14. State two specific manifestations of type V hypersensitivity response?

Answer. The two specific manifestations of type V hypersensitivity responses are Myastenia gravis and Pernicious anemia.

Q15. What are immune complexes?

Answer. Immune complex is the term used to refer to the combination of an antibody with its antigen. Immune complexes must be removed from tissues and kept from accumulating in the circulation and forming deposits throughout the body. Failure to clear immune complexes can lead to autoimmune disease.

Assignments

Q1. List the Coombs and Gell classification for hypersensitivity reactions, give examples of each type?

Q2. Write a short note on the earlier approaches to hypersensitivity?

Q3. Discuss in detail the two phases of DTH?

Q4. Describe stimulatory hypersensitivity and give a specific example?

Q5. Discuss types of immune complex mediated hypersensitivity with their respective examples?

References

Abbas, Abul K, Andrew H. Lichtman, and Shiv Pillai. *Cellular and Molecular Immunology*. Philadelphia: Saunders/Elsevier, 2010. Print.

Ansari, A. A., et al. 1989. Human immune responsiveness to *Lolium perenne* pollen allergen Lol p III (rye III) is associated with HLA-DR3 and DR5. *Hum. Immunol.* **25:**59.

Aubry, J. P., et al. 1992. CD21 is a ligand for CD23 and regulates IgE production. *Nature* **358:**505.

Barnes, K. C., and D. G. Marsh. 1998. The genetics and complexity of allergy and asthma. *Immunol. Today* **19:**325.

Bonnefoy, J. Y., et al. 1993. A new pair of surface molecules involved in human IgE regulation. *Immunol. Today* **14:**1.

Borish, L. 1999. Genetics of allergy and asthma. *Ann. Allergy Asthma Immunol.* **82:**413.

Busse, W., and W. Neaville. 2001. Anti-immunoglobulin E for the treatment of allergic disease. *Curr. Opin. in Allergy & Immunol.* **1:**105.

Chang, T. W. 2000. The pharmacological basis of anti-IgE therapy. *Nat. Biotech.* **18:**157.

Daser, A., et al. 1995. Role and modulation of T-cell cytokines in allergy. *Curr. Opin. Immunol.* **7:**762.

Finkelman, F. D., et al. 1988. IL-4 is required to generate and sustain in vivo IgE response. *J. Immunol.* **141:**2335.

Holt, P. G. 1994. Immunoprophylaxis of atopy: light at the end of the tunnel? *Immunol. Today* **15:**484.

Hoyne, G. F., et al. 1995. Peptide modulation of allergen-specific immune responses. *Curr. Opin. Immunol.* **7:**757.

Kuby Immunology, Judith A. Owen; Jenni Punt; Sharon A. Stranford; Patricia P. Jones; Janis Kuby, New York: W. H. Freeman, ©2013.

Kuhn, R., K. Rajewsky, and W. Muller. 1991. Generation and analysis of interleukin-4 deficient mice. *Science* **254:**707.

Lympany, P., et al. 1992. Genetic analysis of the linkage between chromosome 11q and atopy. *Clin. Exp. Allergy* **22:**1085.

Marsh, D. G., et al. 1994. Linkage analysis of IL-4 and other chromosome 5q31.1 markers and total serum immunoglobulin E concentrations. *Science* **264:**1152.

Marsh, D. G., et al. The Collaborative Study on the Genetics of Asthma (CSGA). 1997. A genome-wide search for asthma susceptibility loci in ethnically diverse populations. *Nat. Genet.* **15:**389.

Metzger, H. 1999. It's spring, and thoughts turn to allergies. *Cell* **97:**287.

Novak, N., S. Kraft, and T. Bieber. 2001. IgE receptors. *Curr. Opinion in Immunol.* **13:**721.

Paul-Eugène, N., et al. 1993. Functional interaction between_2-adrenoceptor agonists and interleukin-4 in the regulation of CD23 expression and release and IgE production in humans. *Molec. Immunol.* **30:**157.

Razin, E., I. Pecht, and J. Rivera. 1995. Signal transduction in the activation of mast cells and basophils. *Immunol. Today* **16:**370.

Roitt's Essential Immunology, Peter J. Delves, Seamus J. Martin, Dennis R. Burton, Ivan M. Roitt. Thirteenth edition. Wiley-Blackwell.

Romagnani, S. 2001. T-cell responses in allergy and asthma. *Curr. Opin. in Allergy & Clin. Immunol.* **1:**73.

Rosenstreich, D. L., et al. 1997. The role of cockroach allergy and exposure to cockroach allergen in causing morbidity among inner-city children with asthma. *N. Engl. J. Med.* **336:**1356.

Russo D., Redman C., Lee S. Association of XK and Kell blood group proteins. *J Biol Chem* 1998; 273:13950–13956.

Schulz D. R., Tozman E. C. Anti-neutrophil cytoplasmic antibodies: major autoantigens, pathophysiology, and disease associations. *Semin Arthritis Rheum* 1995; 25:143–159.

Teixeira, M. M., T. J. Williams, and P. G. Hellewell. 1995. Mechanisms and pharmacological manipulation of eosinophil accumulation. *Trends Pharmacol. Sci.* **16:**418.

Thomas, P., et al. 1992. Glycosylation-inhibiting factor from human T cell hybridomas constructed from peripheral blood lymphocytes of a bee venom–sensitive allergic patient. *J. Immunol.* **148:**729.

Uzzaman A, Cho SH. Classification of hypersensitivity reactions. In *Allergy & Asthma Proceedings* 2012 May 2 (Vol. 33).

Vincent A. Antibody-mediated disorders of neuro-muscular transmission. *Clin Neurophysiol Suppl* 2004; 57:147–158.

Wills-Karp, M., J. Santeliz, and C. L. Karp. 2001. The germless theory of allergic disease: revisiting the hygiene hypothesis. *Nature Rev. Immunol.* **1:**69.

Yamamoto F. I., Clausen H., White T., et al. Molecular genetic basis of the histo-blood group ABO system. *Nature* 1990; 345:229.

Websites

http://www.sciencedirect.com
https://www.ncbi.nlm.nih.gov/pubmed
http://missinglink.ucsf.edu/lm/immunology_module/prologue/
https://www.myvmc.com/diseases/hypersensitivity-reaction
https://www.amboss.com/us/knowledge/Hypersensitivity_reactions

In: The Fundamentals of Hypersensitivities … ISBN: 978-1-53617-012-2
Editor: Manzoor Ahmad Mir

Chapter 3

TYPE I HYPERSENSITIVITY (ALLERGY OR IMMEDIATE TYPE HYPERSENSITIVITY)

Nissar A. Wani, Manzoor Ahmad Mir*, Hina Qayoom, Umar Mehraj, Safura Nisar, Bashir A. Sheikh and Syed Suhail
Department of Bioresources, School of Biological Sciences, University of Kashmir, Srinagar J&K, India

ABSTRACT

These reactions are initiated by the interaction between IgE antibody and a multivalent antigen. IgE antibodies are not alone destructive. Instead they cause hypersensitivity by binding, via their Fc region, to high affinity IgE specific Fc receptors designated FcεRI. FcεRI are expressed by a variety of immune cells like mast cells, basophils and eosinophils. The binding of an antigen to preformed antigen-specific IgE bound to FcεRI initiates type I hypersensitivity reaction. As a result of this cross-linking, mast cells, basophils and eosinophils are stimulated to release their granular contents (histamines, proteases etc.) in a process called, degranulation. Degranulation induces rapid inflammatory response

* Corresponding Author's Email: drmanzoor@kashmiruniversity.ac.in.

(e.g., vasodilation, edema etc.). This ultimately results in clinical manifestations including rhinitis, asthma, and in severe cases anaphylaxis. About 54.3% of the US population suffers from type I hypersensitivity reactions.

Keywords: hypersensitivity type I reaction, IgE, Fc receptors, FcεRI, FcεRII, histamines, leukotrienes, prostaglandins, degranulation, edema

OBJECTIVES

- Understanding how hypersensitivity and allergy result from "mis-direction" of normal adaptive immune responses.
- Outline the importance of the requirement for sensitization prior to reaction.
- Discuss the contributions of various cells (e.g., mast cells and eosinophils) and molecules to normal immune response and to hypersensitivity reactions.
- Describe the common clinical manifestations of different types of hypersensitivities.
- Discuss the means of prevention, evaluation and management of various types of hypersensitivities.

INTRODUCTION

The term hypersensitivity arose from the clinical definition of immunity as "sensitivity" which is based on the observation that an individual who has been exposed to an antigen exhibits a detectable reaction or is "sensitive" to subsequent encounters with that antigen. Thus, hypersensitivity can be defined as a state of increased reactivity to a foreign agent usually acquired by a prior exposure to the same or a chemically related substance. Hypersensitivity reactions require a pre-sensitized state of host. Sensitization, or induction of the hypersensitive state, requires one or more than one exposures to the antigen, followed by a latent period. After the latent period, a reaction is elicited by another exposure to the antigen. The nature of hypersensitivity acquired is determined by the chemical composition of the allergen, the sensitizing route, the physiology and the anatomy of the host and other factors.

TYPES OF HYPERSENSITIVITY REACTIONS

Hypersensitivity reactions are commonly classified according to the type of immune response and the effector mechanism responsible for cell and tissue injury. This classification was originally developed by two British Immunologists, Phillip Gell and Robin Coombs- 1960. According to Coomb-Gell hypersensitivity designations, there are four different types of hypersensitivity reactions:

- Type I hypersensitivity
- Type II hypersensitivity
- Type III hypersensitivity
- Type IV hypersensitivity

Type I Hypersensitivity Reaction (Allergy or Immediate Type Hypersensitivity)

Type I hypersensitivity reaction is commonly known as, "Allergy." Certain types of antigens referred to as, Allergens induce a type I hypersensitive reaction which has all the hallmarks of a normal humoral response. Allergen induces a humoral antibody response in the same way and by the same mechanisms resulting in the generation of antibody secreting plasma cells and memory cells. The difference between a type I hypersensitive response from a normal humoral response is that, the plasma cells secrete Ig E (Figure 3.1).

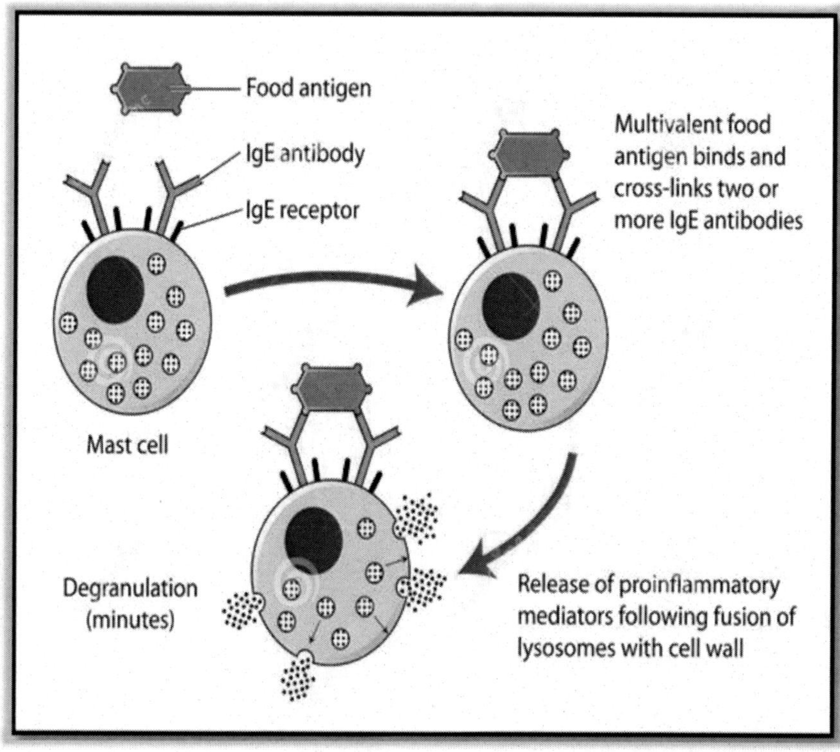

Figure 3.1. Showing the process of degranulation, induced in response to antigen through IgE antibody.

Ig E antibody binds with high affinity to Fc receptors on the surface of mast cells and basophil cells, which contain high levels of biologically active molecules including histamines. On binding of Ig E antibody to mast cells and basophil cells, these cells are said to become sensitized. Later exposure to the same allergen cross-links the membrane-bound Ig E on sensitized mast cells and basophils causing degranulation of these cells. On degranulation the active mediators released from the granules act on the surrounding tissues. The main effects include-vasodilation and smooth-muscle contraction- may be either systemic or localized, depending on the extent of release of active mediators.

COMPONENTS OF TYPE I HYPERSENSITIVITY REACTION

Allergens

The Ig E antibody responses are induced by majority of humans as a defense against parasitic infections. The serum IgE levels increase and remain high until the infection causing parasites are completely removed from the body. Some individuals have an abnormality, which is a hereditary predisposition to the development of immediate hypersensitivity reactions against environmental antigens. This abnormality is called, "Atopy" and the individuals possessing this abnormality are called, Atopic individuals. The Ig E regulatory defects suffered by atopic individuals allow non-parasitic antigens to stimulate inappropriate Ig E production, leading to tissue-damaging type I hypersensitivity.

The term allergen, was first used by "Von Pirquet" to cover all foreign substances that could produce an immune response. Subsequently, the word 'allergen' came to be used selectively for the proteins that cause 'supersensitivity.' Thus, an allergen is an antigen that give rise to immediate hypersensitivity in allergic individuals. The abnormal Ig E response of atopic individuals is partly genetic i.e., it often runs in families. These individuals have abnormally high levels of circulating IgE and more than normal numbers of circulating eosinophils. Atopic individuals are more susceptible to allergies such as, hay fever, eczema and asthma.

It is now known that inherited atopy is multigenic. Most allergic responses occur on mucous membrane surfaces in response to allergens that enter the body by either inhalation or ingestion. Many common allergens have been characterised and purified, which include allergens from rye grass pollen, cod fish, birch pollen, ragweed pollen and bee venom. These allergens have been shown to be a multi-antigenic system that contains a number of allergenic components. It appears that allergenicity is a consequence of a complex series of involving not just the allergen, but also the dose, the sensitising route, sometimes an adjuvant and most important the genetic constitution of the recipient (Table 3.1).

Table 3.1. Some common allergens associated with type I hypersensitivity

Proteins	Vaccines, Foreign serum
Insect products	Bee venom Wasp venom Dust mite Cockroach calyx Ant venom
Foods	Eggs, sea food, Nuts, pears, beans, milk
Plant pollens	Rye grass, Ragweed, Timothy grass, Birch
Mold spores	Animal dander and hair
Drugs	Sulfonamides, Penicillin, salicylates and local anesthetics

Reaginic Antibody (IgE)

The local wheal and flare response that occurs when an allergen is injected into a sensitized individual is called the P-K reaction. It was first demonstrated by K. Prausnitz and H. Kustner in 1921. Because the serum components responsible for the P-K reaction displayed specificity for allergen, they were assumed to be antibodies, but the nature of these P-K antibodies, or reagins, was not demonstrated until many years. In the mid-1960s, the experiments conducted by K. and T. Ishizaka showed that the biological activity of reaginic antibody in a P-K test could be neutralized by rabbit antiserum against whole atopic human sera but not by rabbit antiserum specific for the four human immunoglobulin classes known at that time (IgA, IgG, IgM, and IgD). Furthermore, when rabbits were immunized with sera from ragweed-sensitive individuals, the rabbit antiserum could inhibit (neutralize) a positive ragweed P-K test even after precipitation of the rabbit antibodies specific for the human IgG, IgA, IgM, and IgD isotypes. The Ishizakas called this new isotype IgE in reference to the E antigen of ragweed that they used to characterize it. The serum IgE levels in normal individuals fall within the range of 0.1–0.4 μg/ml; even the most severely allergic individuals rarely have IgE levels greater than 1 μg/ml. These low levels made physiochemical studies of IgE difficult; it was not until the discovery of an IgE myeloma by S. G. O. Johansson and H. Bennich in 1967 that extensive chemical analysis of IgE could be undertaken. IgE was found to be composed of two heavy ε and two light chains with a combined molecular weight of 190,000. The higher molecular weight as compared with IgG (150,000) is due to the presence of an additional constant-region domain. This additional domain (CH4) contributes to an altered conformation of the Fc portion of the molecule that enables it to bind to glycoprotein receptors on the surface of basophils and mast cells. Although the half-life of IgE in the serum is only 2–3 days, once IgE has been bound to its receptor on mast cells and basophils, it is stable in that state for a number of weeks.

IgE-Binding Fc Receptors

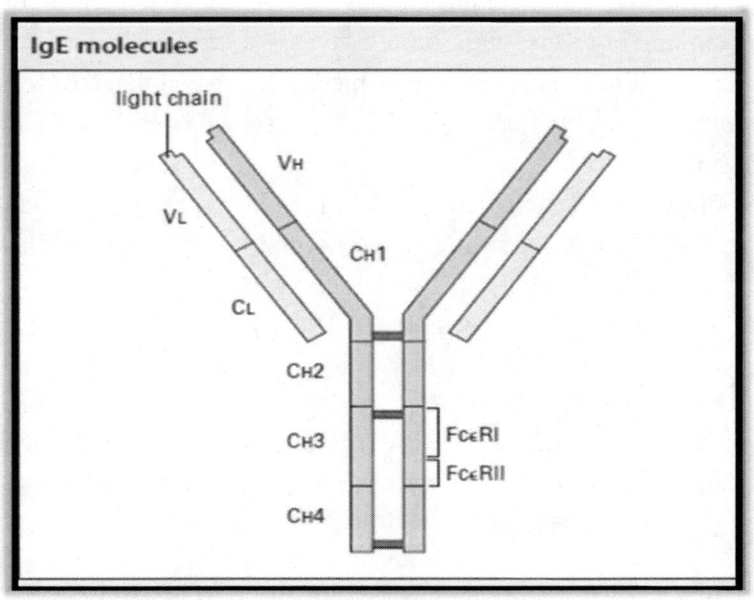

Figure 3.2. The IgE molecule has four heavy chain constant regions. The binding sites for the high-affinity IgE receptor FcεRI and for the low-affinity receptor FcεRII, or CD23, are shown. Monoclonal antibodies to the binding site for FcεRI also block FcεRII.

The reaginic activity of IgE depends on its ability to bind to a receptor specific for the Fc region of the _ heavy chain. Two classes of FcεR been identified, designated FcεRI and FcεRII, which are expressed by different cell types and differ by 1000-fold in their affinity for IgE (Figure 3.2).

Mast cells and basophils express FcεRI, which binds IgE with a high affinity. The high affinity of this receptor enables it to bind IgE despite the low serum concentration of IgE. FcεRI interacts with the CH3/CH3 and CH4/CH4 domains of the IgE molecule via the two Ig-like domains of the α chain. The β-chain spans the plasma membrane four times and is thought to link the α chain to the γ homodimer. The disulfide-linked γ chains extend a considerable distance into the cytoplasm. Each γ chain has a conserved sequence in its cytosolic domain known as an immunoreceptor tyrosine-based activation motif (ITAM). As described earlier, two other membrane receptors that have this motif are CD3 and the associated £ chains of the T-cell receptor complex and the Ig-α/Ig-β chains associated with membrane immunoglobulin on B cells. The ITAM motif on these three receptors interacts with protein tyrosine kinases to transduce an activating signal to the cell. Allergen mediated cross-linkage of the bound IgE results in aggregation of the FcεRI receptors and rapid tyrosine phosphorylation, which initiates the process of mast-cell degranulation. The role of FcεRI in anaphylaxis is confirmed by experiments conducted in mice that lack FcεRI. These mice have normal levels of mast cells but are resistant to localized and systemic anaphylaxis (Figure 3.3).

The other IgE receptor, designated FcεRII (or CD23), is specific for the CH3/CH3 domain of IgE and has a lower affinity for IgE than does FcεRI. The FcεRII receptor appears to play a variety of roles in regulating the intensity of the IgE response. Allergen cross-linkage of IgE bound to FcεRII has been shown to activate B cells, alveolar macrophages, and eosinophils. When this receptor is blocked with monoclonal antibodies, IgE secretion by B cells is diminished. A soluble form of FcεRII (or sCD23), which is generated by autoproteolysis of the membrane receptor, has been shown to enhance IgE production by B cells. Interestingly, atopic individuals have higher levels of CD23 on their lymphocytes and macrophages and higher levels of sCD23 in their serum than do nonatopic individuals.

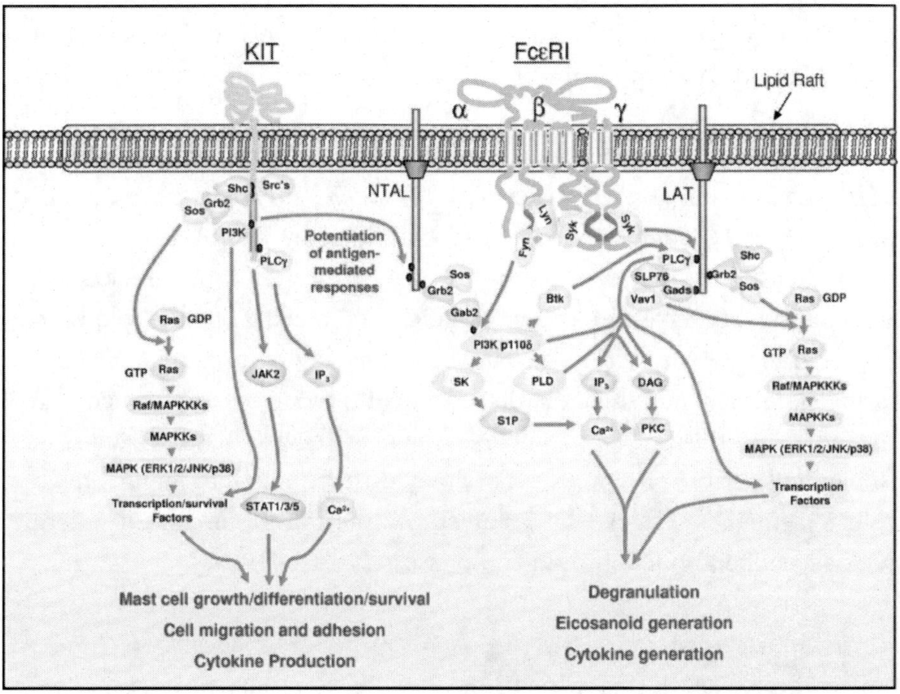

Figure 3.3. Illustrating the kinetics response for induction of IgE mediated response.

Basophils and Mast Cell

Autoradiography revealed that the labeled probe bound IgE has with high affinity to blood basophils and tissue mast cells. Mast cells are found throughout connective tissue, particularly near blood and lymphatic vessels. Some tissues, including the skin and mucous membrane surfaces of the respiratory and gastrointestinal tracts, contain high concentrations of mast cells. Mast cells contain numerous membrane-bounded granules that are distributed throughout the cytoplasm, like those in basophils, which contain pharmacologically active mediators. After activation, these mediators are released from the granules, resulting in the clinical manifestations of the type I hypersensitive reaction. Mast cell populations differ significantly in different anatomic sites in the types and amounts of allergic mediators they contain and in their sensitivity to activating stimuli and cytokines. Mast cells also secrete a large variety of cytokines that affect a broad spectrum of physiologic, immunologic, and pathologic processes.

Basophils are granulocytes that circulate in the blood of most vertebrates; in humans, they account for 0.5%–1.0% of the circulating white blood cells. Their granulated cytoplasm stains with basic dyes, hence the name basophil. Electron microscopy reveals a multilobed nucleus, few mitochondria, numerous glycogen granules, and electron-dense membrane-bound granules scattered throughout the cytoplasm that contain pharmacologically active mediators. Mast-cell precursors are formed in the bone marrow during hematopoiesis and are carried to virtually all vascularized peripheral tissues, where they differentiate into mature cells.

The sequence of events involved in the development of allergic reactions can be divided into several phases:

Sensitization Phase

It is the phase, during which IgE antibody is produced in response to an antigenic stimulus and binds to specific receptors on mast cells and basophils. Healthy individuals produce IgE antibodies only in response to parasitic infections. However, some people, referred to as atopic are genetically predisposed to produce IgE against certain allergens such as plant pollens (e.g., rye grass), food (e.g., nuts), drugs (e.g., penicillin). Allergic reactions can be elicited not only upon re-exposure to same antigen but also to other antigens that have same epitopes. Sensitization to allergens can occur through any means such as skin contact, ingestion, injection and inhalation. Nearly 50% of the population generates IgE response to airborne antigens that are encountered only on mucosal surface such as lining of the nose and lungs and the conjunctiva of the eyes. However, after repeated exposure to a large number of airborne allergens such as plant pollens, mould spores, approximately 20% of the general population develops clinical symptoms resulting in seasonal or perennial allergic rhinitis. Once enough exposure to allergen has been achieved by repeated mucosal contact, ingestion, resulting in the production of IgE antibody, an individual is said to be sensitised (Figure 3.4).

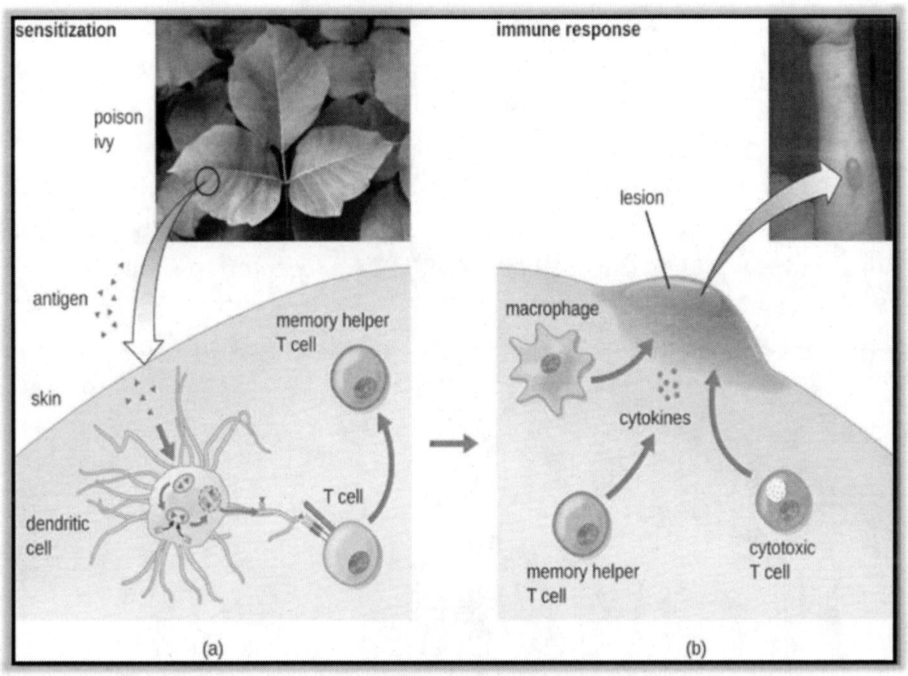

Figure 3.4. (a) On exposure to antigen, the body produces antibodies and memory cells, on repeated exposure an individual is said to be sensitized, (b) Upon re-exposure to the same antigen, the body's memory cells act and generate a response.

Activation Phase

It is the phase, during which re-exposure to the antigen triggers the mast cells and basophils to respond by release of their contents of their granules. At least two of the FcεRI must be bridged together in a stable configuration for the activation phase to occur. This linkage is accomplished by a multivalent antigen that can bind a different molecule of IgE to each of the several epitopes, thus cross linking them on the mast cell surface & triggering the cell to degranulate (Figure 3.5). The physiological consequences of IgE-mediated mast cell degranulation depend on the dose of antigen and route of entry. Mast cells that degranulate within the gastrointestinal tract cause the increased fluid secretion and peristalsis which in turn results in diarrhoea and vomiting. In contrast, degranulation of mast cells in the lung causes a decrease in airway diameters and increased mucous secretion. These events lead to congestion and blockage of airways. Degranulation of mast cells present along the blood vessels causes increased blood flow and vascular permeability, resulting in increased fluid in tissues or edema. This causes increased flow of lymph from the lymph nodes which in turn leads to increased number of cells and increased protein in tissue, all of which contribute to the inflammatory response. Mast cells may also be activated naturally through mechanisms other than IgE Fc receptor cross-linking.

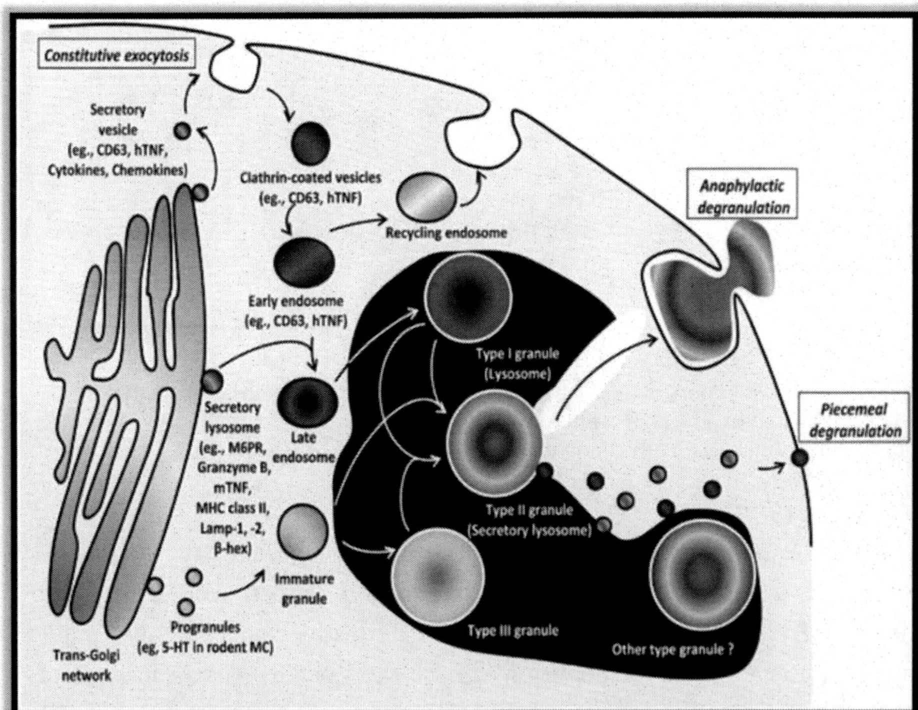

Figure 3.5. Illustrating the mechanism of anaphylactic degranulation.

Anaphylactoid reactions are produced by anaphylatoxins as well as by various drugs like codeine, morphine etc. Physical factors like heat, cold or pressure also activate mast cells for example, cold-induced urticaria is an anaphylactic rash induced in certain individuals by chilling an area of the skin. Another example is dermatographic urticaria in which the skin becomes raised and inflamed when stroked, scratched or slapped.

Effector Phase

It is the phase, during which a complex response occurs as a result of the effects of many inflammatory mediators released by the mast cells and basophils. The symptoms of allergic reactions are entirely attributable to the inflammatory mediators released by the activated mast cells. there are two basic categories of these mediators – preformed mediators which are stored in the granules by electrostatic attraction to a matrix protein and are released as a result of ion influx. Cytokines released from the mast cells including IL-3, IL-4, IL-5, IL-8, IL-9, tumour necrosis factor (TNF)-α and GM-CSF (granulocyte-macrophage-colony stimulating factor) also play an important role in attracting and activating inflammatory cells. The second category, newly synthesised cell mediators, consist of substances synthesised from membrane lipids.

Preformed Mediators

Histamine which is formed by the decarboxylation of the amino acid histidine, is a major component of mast cell granules (Figure 3.6). Its biological effects are observed within minutes of mast cell activation. Once released from mast cells, histamine binds to one of the four different histamine receptors – H_1, H_2, H_3, H_4. This binding induces contraction of the intestinal and bronchial smooth muscles, increased permeability of venules and increased mucous secretion. Interaction of histamine (Figure 3.7) with H_2 receptors increases vasopermeability and vasodilation, stimulates exocrine glands and increases the release of acid in the stomach.

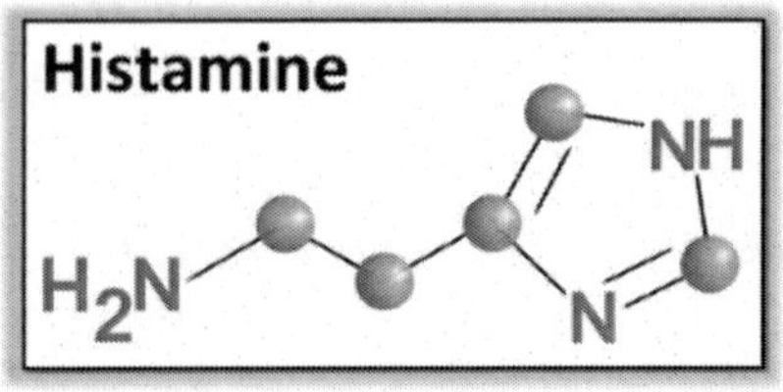

Figure 3.6. Molecular structure of histamine, an active mediator in allergic response.

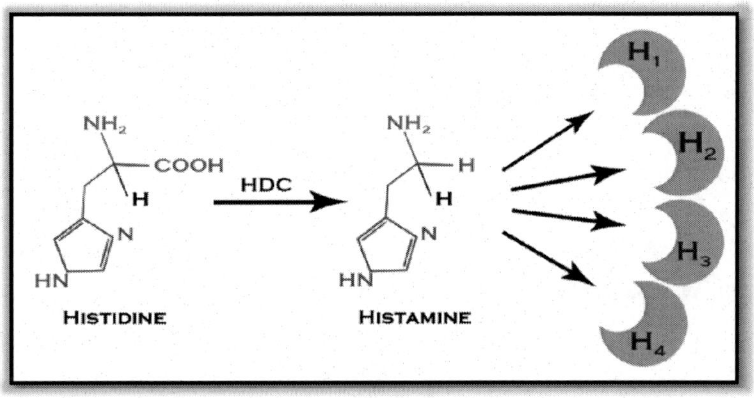

Figure 3.7. Representing the binding of released histamine to four different receptors H1, H2, H3 and H4 on the target cells.

Newly Synthesized Mediators

Leukotrienes and prostaglandins are the secondary mediators and thus are not formed until the mast cell undergoes degranulation and phosholipase signalling initiates the enzymatic breakdown of phospholipids in the plasma membranes.

EARLY AND LATE RESPONSES

Type I hypersensitivity is characterised by both early and late phase responses. The early response occurs within minutes of allergen exposure and results from release of histamine, leukotrienes and prostaglandins from the local mast cells. However, hours after the immediate phase begins to subside, mediators released during the course of reaction induce localised inflammation called the late phase reaction. Cytokines especially TNF-α and IL-1, increase the expression of cell adhesion molecules on venular endothelial cells thus facilitating the influx of neutrophils, eosinophils and T_H2 cells that characterizes this phase.

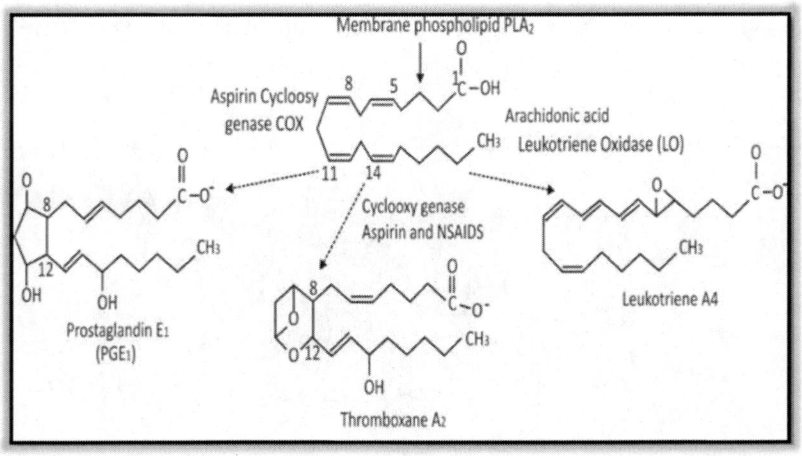

Figure 3.8. Representing the molecular structure of prostaglandins and leukotrienes (secondary mediators in type I hypersensitivity reaction).

Clinical Aspects of Allergic Reactions

The clinical consequences of allergic reactions (atopy) can range from localised reactions (including allergic rhinitis, asthma, atopic dermatitis and food allergies) to severe, life threatening systemic reactions such as anaphylaxis.

Localized Hypersensitivity Reactions

In localised hypersensitivity reactions, the pathology is limited to a specific target tissue or organ. Atopic allergies include a wide range of disorders, such as allergic rhinitis, atopic dermatitis, and food allergies.

- Allergic rhinitis is commonly known as hay fever is the most common atopic disorder worldwide. It is caused by airborne allergens that react with IgE-sensitized mast cells in the nasal passages and conjunctiva (Figure 3.9). Mediators released from the mast cells increase capillary permeability and cause local vasodilation leading to typical symptoms like sneezing and coughing.

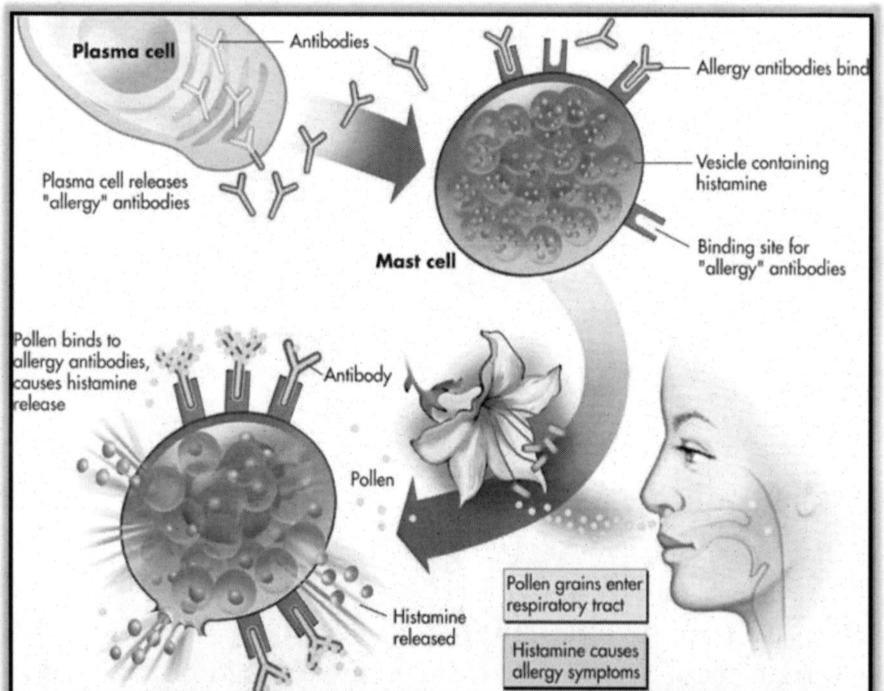

Figure 3.9. Showing the overall process of allergen contact to an individual and release of active effector molecules causing the allergic symptoms.

- Atopic dermatitis or eczema is a form of allergic reaction mostly seen in young children. It is caused by the development of inflammatory skin lesions induced by cytokines. The release of cytokines near the site of allergen contact stimulates chemotaxis of large number of inflammatory cells especially eosinophils (Figure 3.10).

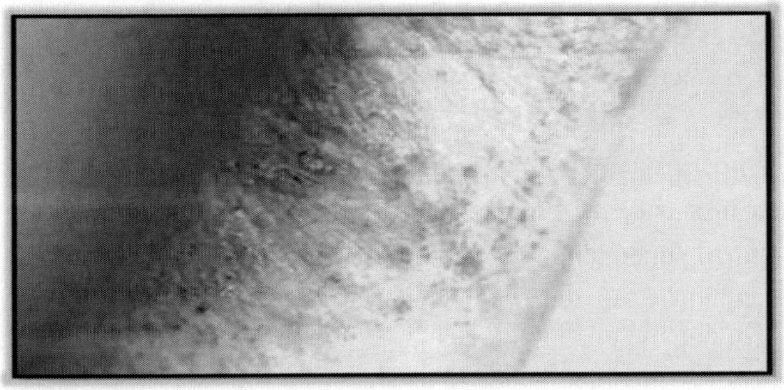

Figure 3.10. Symptoms of atopic dermatitis.

- Food allergies are caused by intake of certain foods e.g., peanuts, rice, eggs, milk etc. ingestion of such foods can trigger the cross linking of allergen specific IgE on mast cells. mast cell degranulation and mediator release leads to localised smooth muscle contraction and vasodilation, often causing vomiting and diarrhoea.
- Asthma is a common form of localised anaphylaxis. It is a chronic disorder of the airways that involves a complex interaction of airflow obstruction, bronchial hyper responsiveness and inflammation. Adhesion molecules antagonists e.g., anti-CAM-1 monoclonal antibodies are being investigated as potential therapies for treatment of asthma. However, corticosteroids remain the gold standard for managing symptoms of asthma.

Systemic Reaction

It includes anaphylaxis which is a shock like, and often fatal state that occurs within minutes of exposure to an allergen. Symptoms include laboured respiration, a precipitous drop in the blood pressure leading to anaphylactic shock followed by contraction of smooth muscles and bronchiolar constriction. This leads to asphyxiation which can lead to death within 2-4 minutes of exposure to the allergen.

DIAGNOSTIC TEST AND TREATMENTS

Type I hypersensitivity is usually assessed by skin-prick test. Small amount of potential allergens is introduced at specific sites on the skin (e.g., forearm or back), either by intradermal injection or by dropping onto the site by a superficial scratch. A positive response to intradermal challenge called *wheal and flare*, is characterised by erythema and edema. More quantitative assays are also available in the laboratory. One such assay, known as the radio allegro sorbent test (RAST) involves covalent coupling of the allergen to the insoluble matrix such as paper discs or beads. The antigen-coated matrix is then dipped into a sample of the patient's serum and allowed to bind any antibody that is specific for the allergen. After the disc is washed, a radiolabelled antibody specific for IgE is added. The amount of radioactivity bound is a measure of the amount of specific IgE antibody in the serum sample (Figure 3.11).

IgE Allergy Testing

Test Type	Diagnostic of IgE Food Allergy	Demonstration of IgE Sensitization
Skin prick testing		
• Scratch or percutaneous testing	No	Yes
• Intradermal	No	Yes
Serological testing		
• sIgE (specific IgE)	No	Yes
• RAST, EIA, Immunocap		
• Component testing	No	Yes
• Microarray	No	Yes
Clinical testing		
Food Challenge	Yes	Yes
Serum IgG	No	No
Atopic Patch testing	No	No
ALCAT (antigen leukocyte antibody test)	No	No

Figure 3.11. Representing various types of test to diagnose different types of allergies. (Source https://slideplayer.com/slide/12552421/)

Sometimes physicians may opt to measure the serum levels of allergen specific IgE using ELISA or western blot techniques.

Treatment of type I hypersensitivity reaction includes avoiding known allergens. Using medications such as steroids and anti-histamines may also help.

Physicians have also been treating allergic patients with repeated exposure of increasing doses of allergens. This regimen is known as hypersensitization or immunotherapy.

CONCLUSION

Type I hypersensitivity also known as, allergic reaction is induced by antigens referred to as allergens. The term allergen refers specifically to non-parasitic antigens capable of stimulating type I hypersensitive responses. Type I hypersensitive reactions are IgE mediated humoral antibody responses. These IgE- mediated reactions are stimulated by the binding of IgE (via; its Fc region) to high affinity IgE-specific Fc receptors expressed on mast cells and basophils. When cross linked by antigens, the IgE antibodies trigger the mast cells and basophils to release primary mediators, vasoactive amines, stored in the granules (degranulation). The most significant primary mediators are histamine, proteases, eosinophil chemotactic factor, neutrophil chemotactic factor and heparin.

These mediators cause all the normal consequences of an acute inflammatory reaction- increased vascular permeability, smooth muscle contraction and extravasation. Mast cell activation via; Fc also leads to the production of two other types of mediators. These secondary mediators, unlike the stored granule contents, must be synthesised de novo and comprise arachidonic acid derivatives (prostaglandins and leukotrienes), platelet-activating factor, and various cytokines.

Type I reaction can be anaphylactic or atopic. Anaphylaxis is a very rapid, life threatening, severe whole body allergic reaction. It is caused by re-exposure to a previously encountered antigen. Atopy (atopic allergy) is a hereditary tendency to develop allergic reaction to substances such as pollen, food, insect venom etc.

MULTIPLE CHOICE QUESTIONS (MCQS)

1. Who gave the classification of hypersensitivity?

A. Robert koch
B. Von pirquet
C. Gell and coomb
D. K-prausnitz and H-kustner

2. Type I hypersensitivity is also known called?

A. Immune complex mediated hypersensitivity
B. Delayed type hypersensitivity
C. Immediate type hypersensitivity
D. Antibody-mediated hypersensitivity

3. The term allergen was given by

A. Gell and coomb
B. K-prausnitz and H-kustner
C. Robert koch
D. Von pirquet

4. The P-K reaction in 1921 was first demonstrated by

A. Robert koch
B. Von pirquet
C. Gell and coomb
D. K-prausnitz and H-kustner

5. Immediate hypersensitivity usually involves

A. mast cells.

B. antibodies to mast cells.

C. platelets.

D. IgG.

6. Mast cell products mediate some of the symptoms of immediate hypersensitivity by increasing

A. IgE receptors.

B. secretion of IgE.

C. capillary leakage.

D. secretion of IgG.

7. Therapy for immediate hypersensitivity includes injection of antigen (allergen) to

A. induce wheal and flare.

B. increase T cells making IL-4.

C. cause anaphylaxis.

D. increase T cells making IFNγ.

8. A hypersensitivity reaction occurs:

A. during the first exposure to an antigen

B. during a second or subsequent exposure to an antigen

C. in individuals with diseases of the immune system

D. Only in children

9. Arrange the following events in the proper order in which they occur during an allergic response.

1. Individual experiences symptoms
2. Individual is sensitized to antigen
3. IgE attaches to mast cells
4. Antigen binds to IgE

A. 1, 2, 3, 4
B. 1, 3, 4, 2
C. 2, 3, 1, 4
D. 2, 3, 4, 1

10. All of the following are associated with type I hypersensitivity except

A. Release of preformed mediators from mast cells
B. Activation of complement
C. Cell-bound antibody bridged by antigen
D. An inherited tendency to respond to allergens

11. To determine if a patient is allergic to rye grass, the best test to perform is

A. Total IgE testing
B. Skin prick test
C. DAT
D. Complement fixation

12. Atopic dermatitis is also often called:

A. Acne
B. Eczema
C. Psoriasis
D. Hives

13. A positive blood test for allergy must include:

A. Antibodies
B. Gluten
C. Antioxidants
D. Enzymes

14. An allergic reaction can produce urticaria. A common term for urticaria is:

A. Atopic dermatitis
B. Eczema
C. Folliculitis
D. Hives

15. Allergies can best be described as:

A. Sneezing, itching, watery eyes, scratchy throat
B. An overreaction from the immune system to a foreign substance
C. The onset of a cold during spring months
D. A reaction to the influenza virus during spring months

ANSWER KEY:

1.C, 2.C, 3.D, 4.D, 5.A, 6.C, 7.D, 8.B, 9.D, 10.B, 11.B, 12.B, 13.A, 14.D, 15.B

FREQUENTLY ASKED QUESTIONS (FAQS)

1. What does hypersensitivity mean?

Answer: The term hypersensitivity arose from the clinical definition of immunity as "sensitivity" which is based on the observation that an individual who has been exposed to an antigen exhibits a detectable.

2. What is allergen? Who gave this term?

Answer: The term allergen, was first used by "Von Pirquet" to cover all foreign substances that could produce an immune response. Subsequently, the word 'allergen' came to be used selectively for the proteins that cause 'supersensitivity.' Thus, an allergen is an antigen that give rise to immediate hypersensitivity in allergic individuals.

3. Differentiate between antigen and allergen?

Answer: Antigen can be any substance (as an immunogen or a hapten) foreign to the body that evokes an immune response either alone or after forming a complex with a larger molecule (as a protein) and that is capable of binding with a product (as an antibody or T cell) of the immune response whereas an allergen is a usually harmless substance capable of triggering a response that starts in the immune system and results in an allergic reaction.

4. What happens when you have an allergic reaction?

Answer: When a person who is allergic to a particular allergen comes into contact with it, an allergic reaction occurs. This begins when the allergen (for example, pollen) enters the body, triggering an antibody response. The antibodies attach themselves to special cells, called mast cells. When the pollen comes into contact with the antibodies, the mast cells respond by releasing certain substances, one of which is called histamine. When the release of histamine is due to an allergen, the resulting swelling and inflammation is extremely irritating and uncomfortable.

5. What is sensitization phase?

Answer: It is the phase, during which IgE antibody is produced in response to an antigenic stimulus and binds to specific receptors on mast cells and basophils. Healthy individuals produce IgE antibodies only in response to parasitic infections. Once enough exposure to allergen has been achieved by repeated mucosal contact, ingestion, resulting in the production of IgE antibody, an individual is said to be sensitised.

6. Define activation phase.

Answer: It is the phase, during which re-exposure to the antigen triggers the mast cells and basophils to respond by release of their contents of their granules. At least two of the FcεRI must be bridged together in a stable configuration for the activation phase to occur. Degranulation of mast cells present along the blood vessels causes increased blood flow and vascular permeability, resulting in increased fluid in tissues or edema. This causes increased flow of lymph from the lymph nodes which in turn leads to increased number of cells and increased protein in tissue, all of which contribute to the inflammatory response.

7. Define effector phase.

Answer: It is the phase, during which a complex response occurs as a result of the effects of many inflammatory mediators released by the mast cells and basophils. The symptoms of allergic reactions are entirely attributable to the inflammatory mediators released by the activated mast cells involving preformed mediators, like histamine which is formed by the decarboxylation of the amino acid histidine, is a major component of mast cell granules and newly synthesized mediators i.e., leukotrienes and prostaglandins that are the secondary mediators and thus are not formed until the mast cell undergoes degranulation and phospholipase signalling initiates the enzymatic breakdown of phospholipids in the plasma membranes.

8. Enumerate the various clinical testing methods for the diagnosis of allergic reactions?

Answer: The probability that a patient has a particular diagnosis can be determined using a combination of diagnostic tests. Some of the allergy tests widely used are:

- Skin prick test
- Patch testing
- Radioallergosorbent test (RAST).

9. What immune cells are involved in immediate hypersensitivity reaction?

Answer: In Type I hypersensitivity response, plasma cells secrete IgE antibodies that bind to mast cells and basophils that then release histamines, a vasodilator, and heparin, a blood thinner.

10. What class of antibody is responsible for immediate hypersensitivity?

Answer: Immunoglobulin E is responsible for immediate hypersensitivity.

11. Discuss the difference between normal immune response to antigen in immunity and in type I hypersensitivity?

Answer: The difference between a normal immune response and a type I hypersensitivity response is that plasma cells secrete IgE antibodies that bind to mast cells and basophils that then release histamines, a vasodilator, and heparin, a blood thinner. This cause inflammation at the site as blood flow to the affected tissues is increased. The reaction may be either local or systemic. Responses usually occur within 30–60 min but can be extremely quick (within minutes) and dramatic as in anaphylaxis.

12. What are the common signs and symptoms seen in hay fever?

Answer: Common symptoms include runny nose and nasal congestion, watery, itchy, red eyes (allergic conjunctivitis), Sneezing, Cough, Itchy nose, fatigue.

13. Are allergies inherited?

Answer: There is a genetic factor involved in the development of allergic disease. If one parent has allergic disease, the estimated risk of a child to develop allergies is 48%; the child's estimated risk grows to 70% if both parents have a history of allergies.

14. Can allergies go away on their own?

Answer: Research has shown that allergic reactions can change over time with age and level of exposure, even disappearing in some cases. However, scientists have not been able to explain as to why and how allergies resolve on their own.

15. Which areas of body may be mostly affected by an allergic reaction?

Answer: Depending on the allergen and where it enters your body, you may experience different symptoms. For example, pollen, when breathed in through the nose, usually causes symptoms in the nose, eyes, sinuses and throat (allergic rhinitis). Allergy to foods usually causes stomach or bowel problems, and may cause hives (urticaria). Allergic reactions can also involve several parts of the body at the same time.

ASSIGNMENTS

Q1. Elucidate the mechanism involved in type I hypersensitivity. Also, discuss the various clinical manifestations.

Q2. Explain the mechanism of pathophysiology of allergic immune response?

Q3. What do you understand by anaphylaxis?

Q4. What are the different diagnostic tests and treatments available for type I hypersensitivity reactions?

Q5. Describe all three phases of type I hypersensitivity.

REFERENCES

Abbas, Abul K, Andrew H. Lichtman, and Shiv Pillai. *Cellular and Molecular Immunology*. Philadelphia: Saunders/Elsevier, 2010. Print.

Beaven MA, Metzger H. Signal transduction by Fc receptors: the FcεRI case. *Immunol Today* 1993;14:222–226.

Borish L, Rosenwasser L. TH1/TH2 lymphocytes: doubt some more. *J Allergy Clin Immunol* 1997;99:161–164.

Bruynzeel-Koomen C, Wichen D, Toonstra J, et al. The presence of IgE molecules on epidermal Langerhans' cells in patients with atopic dermatitis. *Arch Dermatol Res* 1986;278:199–205.

Coca AF, Cooke RA. On the classification of the phenomenon of hypersensitiveness. *J Immunol* 1923;8:163.

Coico, R. and Sunshine, G. (2015). *Immunology: A Short Course*. 7th ed. Wiley-Blackwell.

Coyle AJ, Wagner K, Bertrand C, et al. Central role of immunoglobulin (Ig) E in the induction of lung eosinophil infiltration and T helper 2 cell cytokine production: inhibition by a non-anaphylactogenic anti-IgE antibody. *J Exp Med* 1996;183:1303–1310.

Galli SJ. New concepts about the mast cell. *N Engl J Med* 1993;328:257–265.

Geha RF. Regulation of IgE synthesis in humans. *J Allergy Clin Immunol* 1992;90:143–150.

Haselden BM, Kay AB, Larch M. Immunoglobulin E-independent major histocompatibility complex-restricted T cell peptide epitopeinduced late asthmatic reactions. *J Exp Med* 1999;189:1885–1894.

Kuby Immunology, Judith A Owen; Jenni Punt; Sharon A Stanford; Patricia P Jones; Janis Kuby, New York : W.H. Freeman, ©2013.

Marsh DG, Neely JD, Breezeale DR, et al. Linkage analysis of IL-4 and other chromosome 5q31.1 markers and total serum immunoglobulin E concentrations. *Science* 1994;264:1152-1156.

Miller JS, Schwartz LB. Human mast cell proteases and mast cell heterogeneity. *Curr Opin Immunol* 1989;1:637–642.

Montford S, Robinson HC, Holgate ST. The bronchial epithelium as a target for inflammatory attack in asthma. *Clin Exp Immunol* 1992;22:511–520.

Platts-Mills TAE, Vaughan JW, Squillace S, Woodfolk JA, Sporik RB. Sensitisation, asthma and a modified TH2 response in children exposed to cat allergen. *Lancet* 2001;357:752–756.

Platts-Mills TAE, Vervloet D, Thomas WR, et al. Indoor allergens and asthma: report of the Third International Workshop. *J Allergy Clin Immunol* 1997;100:S2–S24.

Prausnitz C, Kustner H. In: Gell PGH, Coombes RRA, eds. *Clinical aspects of immunology*. Oxford: Blackwell Scientific Publications; 1962:808–816.

Roitt's Essential Immunology, Peter J. Delves, Seamus J. Martin, Dennis R. Burton, Ivan M. Roitt. Thirteenth edition. Wiley-Blackwell.

Sporik R, Holgate ST, Platts-Mills TAE, Cogswell JJ. Exposure to house-dust mite allergen (Der p I) and the development of asthma in childhood. A prospective study. *N Engl J Med* 1990;323:502–507.

Spry CJF, Kay AB, Gleich GJ. Eosinophils 1992. *Immunol Today* 1992;13:384–387.

Wan H, Winton HL, Soeller C, et al. Der p 1 facilitates transepithelial allergen delivery by disruption of tight junctions. *J Clin Invest* 1999;104:123–133.

WAO-White-Book-On-Allregy.pdf.

Wide L, Bennich H, Johansson SGO. Diagnosis of allergy by an in vitro test for allergen antibodies. *Lancet* 1967;ii:1105.

In: The Fundamentals of Hypersensitivities … ISBN: 978-1-53617-012-2
Editor: Manzoor Ahmad Mir

Chapter 4

TYPE II HYPERSENSITIVITY (ANTIBODY-MEDIATED CYTOTOXIC HYPERSENSITIVITY)

Umar Mehraj, Safura Nisar, Bashir A. Sheikh, Syed Suhail, Hina Qayoom and Manzoor Ahmad Mir*
Department of Bioresources, School of Biological Sciences,
University of Kashmir, Srinagar J&K, India

ABSTRACT

Type II hypersensitivity is also known as tissue-specific or cytotoxic hypersensitivity. Type II hypersensitivity is a humoral response mediated by immunoglobulin G or immunoglobulin M that are produced against surface antigens on body cells. Immunoglobulin G and immunoglobulin M antibodies can cause tissue injury by activating the complement system, by recruiting inflammatory cells, and by interfering with normal cellular functions Type II hypersensitivity is mediated by antibodies binding to specific cells. The antibodies damage cells and tissues by activating complement, and by binding and activating effector cells carrying Fcγ receptors. Transfusion reactions to erythrocytes are produced by antibodies to blood group antigens, which may occur naturally or may have been induced by previous contact with incompatible tissue or blood following transplantation, transfusion or during pregnancy. Hemolytic disease of the newborn occurs when maternal antibodies to fetal blood group antigens cross the placenta and destroy the fetal erythrocytes. Type II hypersensitivity reactions may target tissues. Damage to tissues may be produced by antibody to functional cell surface receptors through Fab regions. In doing so, they may enhance or inhibit the normal activity of the receptor. Examples include myasthenia gravis, pemphigus, and Goodpasture's syndrome.

Keywords: Type II hypersensitivity, Ig M, Ig G, Fc receptors, C3 receptors, phagocytosis, transfusion reactions, hemolytic disease

Objectives

- Understand the concept of type II hypersensitivity
- How cells engage their targets using Fc and C3 receptors
- Understand the process how cells damage target cells?
- Discuss the examples of type II hypersensitivity
- Describe effects of transfusion reaction
- Discuss hemolytic disease of new-born
- Describe the drug induced hemolytic anemia

Introduction

Type II hypersensitivity is generally called a tissue-specific, cytolytic, or cytotoxic reaction because it results in the destruction of host cells, either by release of toxic mediators or the lysis. It involves antibody mediated destruction of cells, which is mediated by immunoglobulin G or immunoglobulin M binding to specific cells or tissues. Immunoglobulin G and immunoglobulin M antibodies can cause tissue injury by activating the complement system, by recruiting inflammatory cells, and by interfering with normal cellular functions. Antibody can activate the complement system, creating pores in the membrane of a foreign cell, or it can activate cell destruction by ADCC. The damage caused is therefore, restricted to the specific cells or tissues bearing the antigens. Type II hypersensitivity reaction may occur either by complement-mediated reactions, Antibody-dependent cell-mediated cytotoxicity (ADCC) or Antibody-mediated cellular dysfunction

- *Complement-mediated reactions:* Here the antibodies react with the cell membrane self-antigens. This is followed by complement fixation which activates the complement cascade resulting in the cell lysis. Alternatively, destruction is brought about by opsonisation which ends in phagocytosis.
- *Antibody-dependent cell-mediated cytotoxicity (ADCC):* In this mechanism the cytotoxic cells bearing Fc receptors bind to the Fc region of the antibodies which are already bound to the target cells. The lysis of these cells requires contact but does not involve phagocytosis or complement fixation. Instead, ADCC mediated lysis is analogous to that of cytotoxic T cells and involves release of cytoplasmic granules containing granzymes and perforin. Once released, perforins insert into the target cell and polymerise to form pores. In contrast the granzymes enter the cytoplasm of the target cells and lead to events that cause apoptosis.
- *Antibody-mediated cellular dysfunction:* Sometimes the antibodies bind to the cell surface receptors that are critical for the functional integrity of the cell. When auto-antibodies bind to these receptors they impair or dysregulate the cell function without causing cell injury. Example include, Myasthenia gravis

Cells Bind Their Targets Using Fc and C3 Receptors

In type II hypersensitivity, the cytotoxic (effector) cells with Fc receptors bind to the Fc region of antibodies on target cells and activate complement to bring about damage to the target cells. Antibody bound to a foreign cell also can serve as an opsonin, enabling phagocytic cells with Fc or C3b receptors to bind and phagocytose the antibody-coated cell.

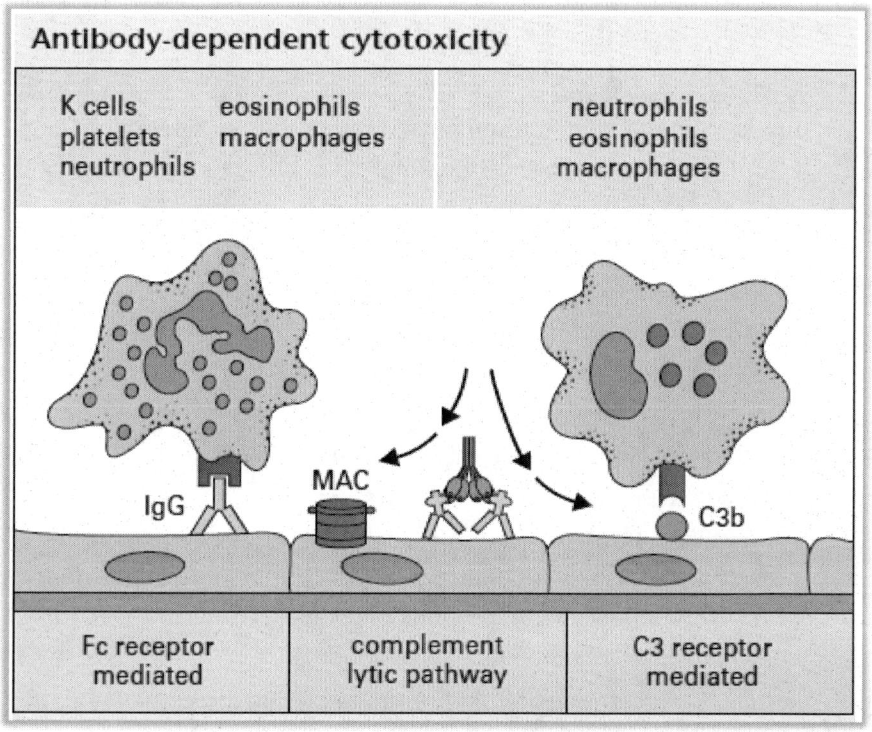

Figure 4.1. Effector cells – K cells, platelets, neutrophils, eosinophils, and cells of the mononuclear phagocyte series – all have receptors for Fc, which they use to engage antibody bound to target tissues. Activation of complement C3 can generate complement-mediated lytic damage to target cells directly, and also allows phagocytic cells to bind to their targets via C3b, C3bi, or C3d, which also activate the cells.(MAC, membrane attack complex).

Once the antibody has attached itself to the surface of the cell or tissue, it can bind and activate compliment component C1, with the following sequences:

- The complement fragments (C3a and C5a) generated by activation of complement attract macrophages and polymorphs to the site, and also stimulate mast cells and basophils to produce chemokines that attract and activate other effector cells

- The classical compliment pathway and activation loop lead to the deposition of C3b, C3bi and C3d, on the target cell membrane;
- The lytic pathway and classical pathway result in the production of the C5b-9 membrane attack complex (MAC) and insertion of the complex into the target cell membrane.

Effector cells- in this case macrophages, neutrophils, eosinophils and NK cells bind to either-the complexed antibody via their Fc receptors; or the membrane bound C3b, C3bi and C3d, via their C3 receptors (CR 1, CR3 and CR4) (Figure 4.1).

Cells Damage Targets by Exocytosis of Their Normal Immune Effector Molecules

The mechanisms by which neutrophils and macrophages damage target cells in type II hypersensitivity reactions reflect their normal methods of dealing with infectious pathogens (Figure 4.2).Normally pathogens would be internalized and then subjected to a barrage of microbicidal systems including defensins, reactive oxygen and nitrogen metabolites, hypohalites, enzymes, altered pH, and other agents that interfere with metabolism. If the target is too large to be phagocytosed, the granule and lysosome contents are released in apposition to the sensitized target in a process referred to as **exocytosis**.

Cross-linking of the Fc and C3 receptors during this process causes activation of the phagocyte with production of reactive oxygen intermediates, as well as activation of phospholipase A2 with consequent release of arachidonic acid from membrane phospholipids. In some situations, such as the eosinophil reaction against schistosomes, exocytosis of granule contents is normal and beneficial. However, when the target is host tissue that has been sensitized by antibody, the result is damaging.

Antibodies may also mediate hypersensitivity by NK cells. In this case, however, the nature of the target, and whether it can inhibit the NK cells' cytotoxic actions, are as important as the presence of the sensitizing antibody. The resistance of a target cell to damage varies. Susceptibility depends on:

- the amount of antigen expressed on the target cell's surface; and
- the inherent ability of different target cells to sustain damage.

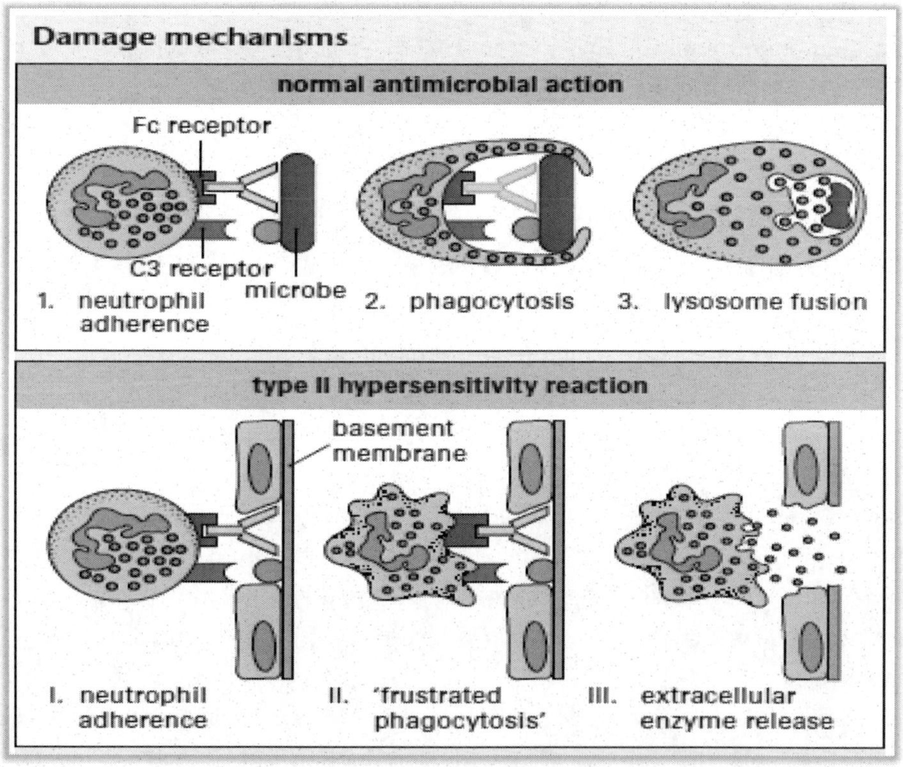

Figure 4.2. Neutrophil-mediated damage is a reflection of normal antibacterial action. (**1**) Neutrophils engage microbes with their Fc and C3 receptors. (**2**) The microbe is then phagocytosed and destroyed as lysosomes fuse to form the phagolysosome (**3**). In type II hypersensitivity reactions, individual host cells coated with antibody may be similarly phagocytosed, but where the target is large, for example a basement membrane (**I**), the neutrophils are frustrated in their attempt at phagocytosis (**II**). They exocytose their lysosomal contents, causing damage to cells in the vicinity (**III**).

For example, an erythrocyte may be lyzed by a single active C5 convertase site, whereas it takes many such sites to destroy most nucleated cells – their ion-pumping capacity and ability to maintain membrane integrity with anti-complementary defenses is so much greater.

Examples of Type II Hypersensitivity Reactions

Some of the instances where type II hypersensitivity reactions are thought to be of prime importance in causing target cell destruction or immunopathological damage are:

- Transfusion reactions
- Hemolytic disease of the new-born
- Drug-induced hemolytic anemia

Transfusion Reactions Are Type II Hypersensitivity Reactions

Within each system there may be two or more phenotypes. In the ABO system, for example, there are four phenotypes (A, B, AB, and O), and therefore four possible blood groups encoded by the different genes, each of which has a number of alternative alleles. An individual possessing one allelic form of a blood group antigen can recognize other allelic forms of an transfused blood as foreign and mount an antibody response. However, for some blood group antigens such antibodies can also be produced 'naturally' (i.e., without previous sensitization by foreign erythrocytes) by natural exposure to similar antigenic determinants on a variety of microorganisms present in the normal flora of the gut.

Antibodies to the A,B and O antigens, called Isohemagglutinins are usually of the class Ig M and cause agglutination, compliment activation and intravascular hemolysis. A person with blood type A, e.g; recognises B-like antigens on intestinal microorganisms and produces

Isohemagglutinins to the B-like antigens. This same person on exposure to A-like antigen on the same intestinal microorganism doesn't respond because these A-like antigens are too similar to self and a state of self-tolerance to these antigens should exist.

If an individual with type A blood is transfused with blood containing type B cells, a transfusion reaction occurs in which the anti-B Isohemagglutinins bind to the B blood cells and mediate their destruction by the means of compliment mediated lysis (Table 4.1).

Table 4.1. Representing ABO genotypes and corresponding phenotypes, agglutinins and isohemagglutinins

Genotype	Blood-group phenotype	Antigens on erythrocytes (agglutinins)	Serum antibodies (Isohemagglutinins)
AA or AO	A	A	Anti-B
BB or BO	B	B	Anti-A
AB	AB	A and B	None
OO	O	None	Anti-A and anti-B

The clinical manifestations of transfusion reaction result from intravascular hemolysis of the transfused red blood cells by antibody plus compliment.

These manifestations may be either immediate or delayed. Reactions that begin immediately are most commonly associated with ABO blood group incompatibilities which lead to compliment mediated lysis triggered by the Ig M Isohemagglutinins. Free hemoglobin can be detected within hours in the plasma, through kidneys it is filtered, resulting in the *hemoglobinuria.* Some of the hemoglobin gets converted to bilirubin, which at high levels is toxic.

Symptoms include fever, clotting in blood vessels, nausea, hemoglobin in the urine, lower back pain, chills. Its treatment involves termination of the transfusion and maintenance of urine flow with diuretic, because accumulation of hemoglobin in the kidney can cause acute tubular necrosis.

Table 4.2. Not all blood groups are equally antigenic in transfusion reactions – thus RhD evokes a stronger reaction in an incompatible recipient than the other Rhesus antigens; and Fy^a is stronger than Fyb. Frequencies stated are for Caucasian populations- other races have different gene frequencies

System	Gene loci	Antigens	Phenotype frequency (%)	
ABO	1	A, B, or O	A	42
			B	8
			AB	3
			O	47
Rhesus	2 closely linked loci: major antigen=RhD	C or c	RhD$^+$	85
		D or d	RhD$^-$	15
		E or e		
Kell	1	K or k	K	9
			K	91
Duffy	1	FY^a, Fy^b or Fy	FY^a Fy^b	46
			FY^a	20
			Fy^b	34
			FY	0.1
MN	1	M or N	M	28
			MN	50
			NN	22

Antibodies to other blood group antigens may result from repeated blood transfusions i.e; delayed hemolytic transfusion reaction. It generally occurs in individuals who have received repeated transfusions of ABO-compatible blood that is incompatible for other blood group antigens. The reaction develop between 2 and 6 days after transfusion, reflecting the secondary nature of these reactions. The transfused blood induces clonal selection and production of Ig G against a variety of blood group membrane antigens, most commonly Rh, Kell, Duffy, Kidd because minor allelic differences in these antigens can stimulate antibody production (Table 4.2). These antibodies are of the class Ig G, which cause less agglutination than Ig M. The Ig G sensitized cells are usually taken up by phagocytes in the liver and spleen, through severe reactions may cause erythrocyte destruction by compliment activation. This can cause circulatory shock and the released contents of the erythrocytes can produce acute tubular necrosis of the kidneys. These transfusion reactions are often seen in previously unsensitized individuals and develop over days or weeks as antibodies to the foreign cells are produced. This can result in anemia or jaundice.

Transfusion of allogeneic erythrocytes into an individual who already has antibodies against them may produce erythrocyte destruction and symptoms of a 'transfusion reaction'. Some blood group systems (e.g., ABO and Rhesus) are characterized by antigens that are relatively strong immunogens; such antigens are more likely to induce antibodies. When planning a blood transfusion, it is important to ensure that donor and recipient blood types are compatible with respect to these major blood groups, otherwise transfusion reactions will occur.

HDNB (Hemolytic Disease of the New-Born) Is Caused by Type II Hypersensitivity Reactions

Hemolytic disease of the newborn (HDNB) occurs when the mother has been sensitized to antigens on the infant's erythrocytes and makes IgG antibodies specific for fetal blood group antigens. These antibodies cross the placenta and react with the fetal erythrocytes, causing destruction of fetal red blood cells. The consequences of such transfer can be minor, serious or lethal. Rhesus D (RhD) is the most commonly involved antigen. Erythroblastosis fetalis, a severe hemolytic disease of the new-born, most commonly develops when a Rh+-sensitized Rh− mother carries a second Rh+ infant. Sensitization of the Rh− mother to the Rh+ erythrocytes usually occurs during the birth of the first Rh+ infant, when some fetal erythrocytes leak back across the placenta at the time of delivery into the maternal circulation and are recognized by the maternal immune system. These fetal red blood cells activate Rh specific B cells, resulting in the production of Rh-specific plasma cells and memory B cells in the mother.

During her first pregnancy with a Rh+ fetus, an Rh− woman is usually not exposed to enough fetal red blood cells to activate her Rh− specific B cells (Figure 4.3). The first incompatible child is therefore usually unaffected, whereas subsequent children have an increasing risk of being affected, as the mother is re-sensitized with each successive pregnancy because the secreted Ig M antibody clears the Rh+ fetal red cells from the mother's circulation, but the memory cells remain a threat to any subsequent pregnancy with an Rh+ fetus. In a subsequent pregnancy, activation of these memory cells results in the formation of Ig G anti-Rh antibodies, which cross the placenta and destroy the fetal red blood cells. It may result in mild to severe anemia can develop in the fetus, sometimes with fatal consequences. Furthermore, Conversion of hemoglobin to bilirubin can present another threat to the infant as the lipid-soluble bilirubin may accumulate in the brain and lead to brain damage.

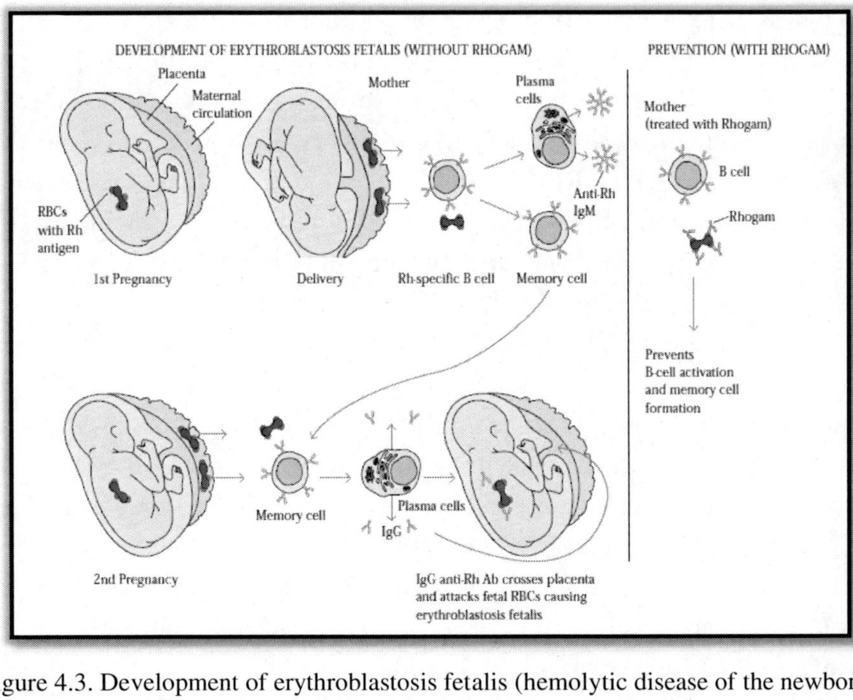

Figure 4.3. Development of erythroblastosis fetalis (hemolytic disease of the newborn) caused when an Rh– mother carries an Rh+ fetus (*left*), and effect of treatment with anti-Rh antibody, or Rhogam(*right*).

Reactions to other blood groups may also cause HDNB, the second most common being the Kell system K antigen. Reactions due to anti-K are much less common than reactions due to RhD because of the relatively low frequency (9%) and weaker antigenicity of the K antigen. Hemolytic disease of the new-born caused by Rh-incompatibility in a subsequent pregnancy can be almost entirely prevented by administering antibodies against the Rh antigen to the mother within 24-48 hours after the first delivery. These antibodies called, Rhogam, bind to any fetal red blood cells that enter the mother's circulation during birth of the first baby and facilitate their clearance before B-cell activation ensuring no memory cell production.

The risk of HDNB due to Rhesus incompatibility is known to be reduced if the father is of a different ABO group to the mother. This observation led to the idea that these Rh− mothers were destroying Rh+ cells more rapidly because they were also ABO incompatible. Consequently, fetal Rh+ erythrocytes would not be available to sensitize the maternal immune system to RhD antigen. This notion led to the development of *Rhesus prophylaxis* – preformed anti-RhD antibodies are given to Rh− mothers immediately after delivery of Rh+ infants, with the aim of destroying fetal Rh+ erythrocytes before they can cause Rh− sensitization. This practice has successfully reduced the incidence of HDNB due to Rhesus incompatibility Although the number of cases of HDNB has fallen dramatically and progressively, the proportion of cases caused by other blood groups, including Kell and the ABO system, has increased

If Rh-incompatibility is detected during pregnancy presenting a threat of hemolytic disease, the treatment depends on the severity of the reaction. In more severe cases, the fetus can be given an intrauterine blood exchange transfusions to replace fetal Rh+ red blood cells with Rh−cells, after every 10-21 days until delivery. In less severe cases, a blood exchange transfusions is not given until after birth, to remove bilrubin; the infant is also exposed to low levels of UV light to breakdown the bilrubin and prevent cerebral damage.

The mothers can be treated during the pregnancy by plasmopheresis. Type A or B fetuses carried by type O mothers most commonly develop these reactions. A type O mother is likely to develop Ig G class of antibody to the A or B blood group antigens either through natural exposure or through exposure to fetal-blood group A or B epitopes in successive pregnancies.

The development of hemolytic disease of the newborn caused by Rh incompatibility can be detected by testing maternal serum at intervals during pregnancy for antibodies to the Rh antigen. A rise in the titer of these antibodies as pregnancy progresses indicates that the mother has been exposed to Rh antigens and is producing increasing amounts of antibody. The presence of maternal IgG on the surface of fetal red blood cells can be detected by a Coombs test. Isolated fetal red blood cells are incubated with the Coombs reagent, goat antibody to human IgG antibody. If maternal IgG is bound to the fetal red blood cells, the cells agglutinate with the Coombs reagent.(Figure 4.4)

DRUG-INDUCED HEMOLYTIC ANEMIA IS A TYPE II HYPERSENSITIVITY REACTION

Certain antibiotics (e.g., penicillin, cephalosporin, and streptomycin) can adsorb nonspecifically to proteins on RBC membranes, forming a complex similar to a hapten-carrier complex. In some patients, such drug-protein complexes induce formation of antibodies, which then bind to the adsorbed drug on red blood cells, inducing complement mediated lysis and thus progressive anemia. When the drug is withdrawn, the hemolytic anemia disappears. Penicillin is notable in that it can induce all four types of hypersensitivity with various clinical manifestations.

Drugs (or their metabolites) can provoke hypersensitivity reactions against blood cells, including erythrocytes and platelets. This can occur in three different ways.

- Hemolytic anemias have been reported following the administration of a wide variety of drugs, including:

  - penicillin;
  - quinine; and
  - sulfonamides.

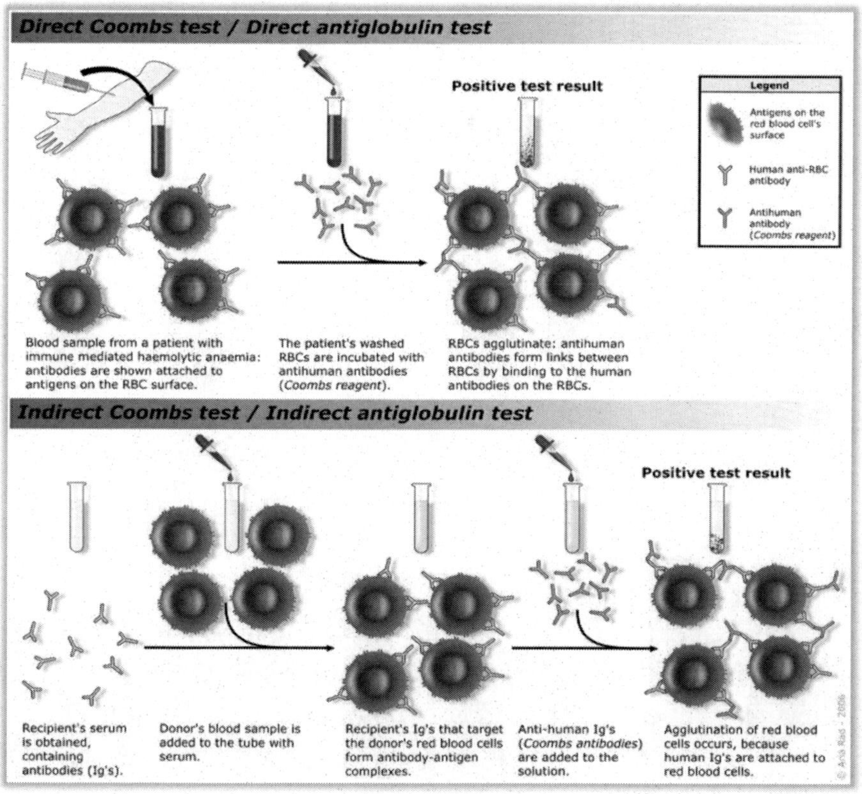

Figure 4.4. This test, also called a Coombs' test, is used to detect antibody on a patient's erythrocytes. If antibody is present the erythrocytes can be agglutinated by anti-human immunoglobulin. If no antibody is present on the red cells, they are not agglutinated by anti-human immunoglobulin.

- The drug binds to the blood cells and antibodies are produced against the drug – In this case it is necessary for both the drug and the antibody to be present to produce the reaction. This phenomenon was first recorded by Ackroyd, who noted thrombocytopenic purpura (destruction of platelets leading to purpuric rash) following administration of the drug Sedormid.

All these conditions are rare.

- Drug–antibody immune complexes are adsorbed onto the erythrocyte cell membrane – When drug–antibody immune complexes are adsorbed on to the erythrocyte cell membrane damage occurs by complement mediated lysis (Figure 4.5).

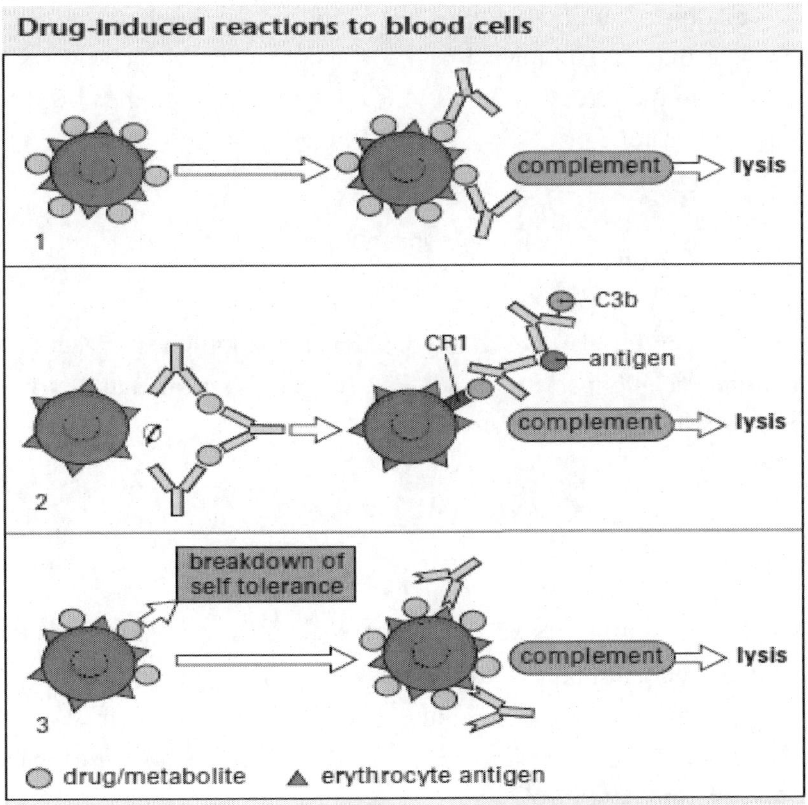

Figure 4.5. Three ways that drug treatment can cause damage are illustrated. (**1**) The drug adsorbs to cell membranes. Antibodies to the drug bind to the cell and complement mediated lysis occurs. (**2**) Immune complexes of drugs and antibody become adsorbed to the red cell. This could be mediated by an Fc receptor, but is more probably via the C3b receptor CR1. Damage occurs by complement-mediated lysis. (**3**)

- The drug induces an allergic reaction – The drug induces an allergic reaction and autoantibodies are directed against the erythrocyte antigens themselves, as occurs in 0.3% of patients given a-methyldopa. The antibodies produced are similar to those in patients with warm-reactive antibody. However, the condition remits shortly after the cessation of drug treatment

Drugs, presumably adsorbed onto cell membranes, induce a breakdown of self-tolerance, possibly by stimulating TH cells. This leads to the formation of antibodies to other blood group antigens on the cell surface. Note that in examples 1 and 2 the drug must be present for cell damage to occur, whereas in 3 the cells are destroyed whether they carry adsorbed drug or not.

Myasthenia Gravis

In this condition the antagonistic autoantibodies reactive to acetylcholine receptors in the motor end plate of skeletal muscles impair neuromuscular transmission, causing muscle weakness.

Graves' Disease

Here the autoantibodies serve as agonists causing stimulation of target cells. these autoantibodies are targeted against thyroid-stimulating hormone receptor on the thyroid epithelial cells, causing hyperthyroidism.

Other examples of type II hypersensitivity reactions are Good pasture syndrome, Thrombocytopenia etc.

CONCLUSION

Type II hypersensitivity reaction is generally called a cytolytic or cytotoxic reaction because it results in the destruction of host cells, either by lysis or toxic mediators. Type II hypersensitivity is caused by antibodies binding to cells or tissue antigens. The antibodies are of the IgM or IgG classes and cause cell destruction by Fc dependent mechanisms either directly or by recruiting complement via the classical pathway. Classical examples of type II hypersensitivity reactions are the response exhibited by a person who receives a transfusion with blood from a donor with a different blood group and erythroblastosis fetalis. Two different antibody-mediated mechanisms are involved in these reactions. In "complement-mediated hypersensitivity reactions", the antibodies react with a cell membrane component, leading to complement fixation. This activates the compliment cascade and leads either to lysis of the cell or opsonization. Blood cells are most commonly affected by this mechanism. "ADCC" used Fc receptors expressed on many cell types (e.g., natural killer cells, macrophages, eosinophils, neutrophils) as a means of bringing these cells into contact with antibody-coated target cells. Lysis of these target cells requires contact but doesn't involve phagocytosis or complement fixation. Instead, ADCC lysis of target cells is analogous to that of cytotoxic T cells and involves the release of cytoplasmic granules containing perforin and granzymes that activate events leading to apoptosis. ADCC reactions involve IgG and IgG Fc receptors.

MULTIPLE CHOICE QUESTIONS (MCQS)

1. A transfusion reaction (ABO incompatible blood) is found to be specific manifestation of:

A. Type I hypersensitivity
B. Type II hypersensitivity
C. Type III hypersensitivity
D. Type IV hypersensitivity

2. Which of the following type of hypersensitivity is also called "antibody-mediated hypersensitivity"?

A. Type I hypersensitivity
B. Type II hypersensitivity
C. Type III hypersensitivity
D. Type IV hypersensitivity

3. Graves' disease is an example of _______ hypersensitivity.

A. Type I hypersensitivity
B. Type II hypersensitivity
C. Type III hypersensitivity
D. Type IV hypersensitivity

4. The principal antibodies involved in type II hypersensitivity are:

A. IgD and IgM
B. IgG and IgM
C. IgG and IgE
D. IgA and IgD

5. Antibody dependent cytotoxicity is associated with

A. Type I hypersensitivity
B. Type II hypersensitivity
C. Type III hypersensitivity
D. Type IV hypersensitivity

6. Goodpasture's disease involving lesions in the kidney and in lung alveoli is caused by

A. deposition of soluble antigen–antibody complexes.
B. cell mediated hypersensitivity to kidney antigens.
C. IgE antibodies to proximal tubules.
D. antibodies to basement membranes.
E. non-specific reactions due to a high level of serum IgG.

7. Complement receptors on red blood cells and Fc receptors on platelets probably facilitate

A. immune phagocytosis of immune complexes by red blood cells and platelets.
B. immune pinocytosis of immune complexes by red blood cells and platelets.
C. the synthesis of gamma interferon by the platelet.
D. the elimination of immune complexes by phagocytic cells.

8. Hemolytic disease of the newborn due to RhD incompatibility depends upon the

A. mother possessing RhD antigens not present on the baby's red cells.
B. inability of the baby to react against the mother's red cells.
C. transplacental passage of IgM anti-RhD antibodies.
D. transplacental passage of IgG anti-RhD antibodies.
E. production of cytotoxic antibodies by the baby.

9. Anti-RhD antibody

A. is not given to RhD negative mothers after birth of an RhD positive infant.
B. does not react with RhD antigens on RBC.
C. does not block the development of active immunity to RhD antigen.
D. is obtained from RhD negative women.

10. Newborns

A. receive IgM antibodies from the mother through placental transfer.
B. have virtually a full complement of maternal IgG antibodies.
C. have very few lymphocytes in their circulation.
D. respond to antigens as well as adults.
E. receive maternal B cells.

11. Antibody dependent cell mediated cytotoxicity (ADCC)

A. is carried out by B cells.
B. is the main mechanism for killing intracellular microbes.
C. involves Fc receptors on the effector cells.
D. is primarily mediated by IgE antibody.

12. Human IgM

A. crosses the placenta.
B. consists of 3 subunits linked together by a J chain.
C. protects mucosal surfaces.
D. is largely restricted to the circulation.
E. is the antibody produced by high affinity plasma cells.

13. A B cell can express on its cell surface

A. membrane IgM and IgD at the same time.
B. both types of light chain.
C. secretory component.
D. IgG that can bind several different unrelated antigens.

14. The major immunoglobulin class found in colostrum is

A. IgG.
B. IgA.
C. IgM.
D. IgE.
E. IgD.

15. Immunosuppression is not induced by

A. antihistamines.
B. removal of lymphoid tissue.
C. use of anti-lymphocyte antibodies.
D. cytotoxic drugs.

ANSWER KEY:

1.B, 2.B, 3.B, 4.B, 5.B, 6.D, 7.D, 8.D, 9.D, 10.B, 11.C, 12.D, 13.A, 14.B, 15.A

FREQUENTLY ASKED QUESTIONS (FAQS)

1. Define cytotoxic hypersensitivity?

Answer: Type II hypersensitivity is also known as tissue-specific or cytotoxic hypersensitivity. Type II hypersensitivity is a humoral response mediated by immunoglobulin G or immunoglobulin M that are produced against surface antigens on body cells

2. Outline the course of process of opsonization in hypersensitivity type II reaction?

Answer: The process of opsonization in hypersensitivity type II reaction occurs by three pathways viz,

- Phagocytosis: First the immunoglobulin G or immunoglobulin M antibodies coating target cells can bind to Fc receptors present on cells such as macrophages and neutrophils and mediate phagocytosis.
- Complement dependent cytotoxicity: Immunoglobulin G or immunoglobulin M antibodies can also activate complement system via the classical pathway. Complement activation leads to the production of Membrane Attack Complexes, which forms pores in cellular membranes resulting in cytolysis (CDC).
- Antibody dependent cellular cytotoxicity (ADCC): A quite distinct cytotoxic mechanism, antibody dependent cellular cytotoxicity (ADCC) occurs when target cells coated with antibody are killed through an extra-cellular non-phagocytic process involving leukocytes that bind to the target by their specific Fc receptors.

3. Give three examples of type II hypersensitivity reaction.

Answer: Some of the instances where type II hypersensitivity reactions are thought to be of prime importance is in causing target cell destruction or immunopathological damage. The following three examples of type II hypersensitivity are:

- Transfusion reactions
- Hemolytic disease of the new-born
- Drug-induced hemolytic anemia

4. What do you mean by transfusion reactions?

Answer: If an individual with type A blood is transfused with blood containing type B cells, a transfusion reaction occurs in which the anti-B Isohemagglutinins bind to the B blood cells and mediate their destruction by the means of compliment mediated lysis.

5. Describe some of the symptoms induced by transfused reactions.

Answer: Some typical symptoms induced by transfused reactions are: fever, chills, nausea, clotting with in blood cells, pain in lower back and hemoglobin in urine.

6. Which antibodies are associated with ABO blood group incompatibilities and a variety of other blood group membrane antigens?

Answer: IgM antibodies are commonly associated with ABO blood group incompatibilities, which lead to complement-mediated lysis and IgG antibodies are associated with Rh, Kidd, Kell and Duffy blood-membrane antigens.

7. What is hemolytic disease?

Answer: Hemolytic disease of the newborn (HDNB) occurs when the mother has been sensitized to antigens on the infant's erythrocytes and makes IgG antibodies specific for fetal blood group antigens. These antibodies cross the placenta and react with the fetal erythrocytes, causing destruction of fetal red blood cells. The consequences of such transfer can be minor, serious or lethal.

8. How can hemolytic disease of the new born be diagnosed?

Answer: Hemolytic disease of the new born caused by Rh-incompatibility in a subsequent pregnancy can be almost entirely prevented by administering antibodies against the Rh antigen to the mother within 24-48 h after the first delivery. These antibodies called, Rhogam, bind to any fetal red blood cells that enter the mother's circulation at the time of delivery and facilitate their clearance before B-cell activation and ensuring memory cell production can't take place.

9. How can the HDNB (hemolytic disease of the new born) be detected?

Answer: The development of hemolytic disease of the new born caused by Rh-incompatibility can be detected by testing maternal serum at intervals during pregnancy for antibodies to the Rh antigen. A rise in the titer of these antibodies as pregnancy progresses indicates that the mother has been exposed to Rh antigens and is producing increasing amounts of antibody.

10. Which antibody is involved in type II hypersensitivity reaction?

Answer: IgG and IgM are the two antibodies involved in generating type II hypersensitivity response.

11. Explain the Coomb's test.

Answer: The presence of maternal Ig G on the surface of fetal red blood cells can be detected by Coomb's test. Isolated fetal red blood cells are incubated with Coomb's reagent, goat antibody to human IgG antibody. If maternal IgG is bound to the fetal red blood cells, the cells agglutinate with the Coomb's reagent. If hemolytic disease caused by Rh-incompatibility is detected during pregnancy, the treatment depends on the severity of the reaction.

12. Explain the effects of Rh-incompatibility between the mother and the fetus.

Answer: Severe hemolytic disease of the new born, called erythroblastosis fetalis, most commonly develops when an Rh+ fetus expresses an Rh antigen on its blood cells that the Rh- mother does not express. During pregnancy, fetal red blood cells are separated from the mother's circulation by a layer of cells in the placenta called, the trophoblast. Mild to severe anemia can develop in the fetus, sometimes with fatal consequences. In addition, conversion of hemoglobin to bilrubin can present an additional threat to the new born because the lipid-soluble bilrubin may accumulate in the brain and cause brain damage.

13. How can the accumulated bilrubin in the new born be removed?

Answer: In less severe cases, a blood-exchange transfusion is not given until after birth, primarily to remove bilrubin, the infant is also exposed to low levels of UV light to breakdown the bilrubin and prevent cerebral damage.

14. How drugs induce hemolytic anemia?

Answer: Certain antibodies can absorb non-specifically to proteins on RBC membranes, forming a complex similar to a haten-carrier complex. In some patients, such drug-protein complexes induce formation of antibodies, which then bind to the adsorbed drug on red blood cells, inducing complement-mediated lysis and thus progressive anemia. When the drug is withdrawn, the hemolytic anemia disappears.

15. Name some of the drugs responsible for the drug-induced hemolytic anemia.

Answer: Penicillin, streptomycin and cephalosporin are some of the drugs responsible for causing drug-induced hemolytic anemia

ASSIGNMENTS

Q1. Briefly describe the mechanism involved in antibody-dependent cell-mediated cytotoxicity (ADCC).

Q2. Explain antibody-mediated cytotoxic hypersensitivity.

Q3. Describe the effects of hemolytic anemia.

Q4. Pen down the features of phagocytosis.

Q5. Find the mechanism of how and which drugs induce hemolytic anemia.

REFERENCES

Abbas, Abul K, Andrew H. Lichtman, and Shiv Pillai. *Cellular and Molecular Immunology*. Philadelphia: Saunders/Elsevier, 2010. Print.

Alarçon-Segovia D, Ruiz-Argüelles A, Llorente L. Broken dogma: penetration of autoantibodies into living cells. *Immunol Today* 1996;17:163-164.

Amagai M. Autoantibodies against desmosomal cadherins in pemphigus. *J Dermatol Sci* 1999;20:92–102.

Anstee DJ. *Blood group active substances of the human red blood cell.* Vox Sang 1990;58:1.

Bhol K, Natarajan K, Nagarwalla N, et al. Correlation of peptide specificity and IgG subclass with pathogenic and non-pathogenic auto-antibodies in pemphigus vulgaris: a model for autoimmunity. *Proc Natl Acad Sci USA* 1995;92:5239–5243.

Black M, Mignogna MD, Scully C. Pemphigus vulgaris. *Oral Dis* 2005;11:119–130.

Bloy C, Blanchard D, Lambin P, et al. Characterization of the D, C, E and G antigens of the Rh blood group system with human monoclonal antibodies. *Mol Immunol* 1988;25:926–930.

Coico, R. and Sunshine, G. (2015). *Immunology: A Short Course*. 7th ed. Wiley-Blackwell.

Dean FG, Wilson GR, Li M, Edgtton KL, et al. Experimental autoimmune Goodpasture's disease: a pathogenetic role for both effector cells and antibody injury. *Kidney Int* 2005;67:566–575.

Demoly P, Hillaire-Buys D. Classification and epidemiology of hypersensitivity drug reactions. *Immunology and Allergy Clinics.* 2004 Aug 1;24(3):345-56.

Descotes J, Choquet-Kastylevsky G. Gell and Coombs's classification: Is it still valid?. *Toxicology.* 2001 Feb 2;158(1-2):43-9.

Druet P, Glotz D. Experimental autoimmune nephropathies: induction and regulation. *Adv Nephrol* 1984;13:115.

Engelfriet CP, Reesink HW, Judd WJ, et al. Current status of immunoprophylaxis with anti-D immunoglobulin. *Vox Sang* 2003;85:328–337.

King MJ. Blood group antigens on human erythrocytes –distribution, structure and possible functions. *Biochim Biophys Acta* 1994;1197:14–44.

Kuby Immunology, Judith A Owen; Jenni Punt; Sharon A Stranford; Patricia P Jones; Janis Kuby, New York: W.H. Freeman, ©2013

Lang B, Newsom-Davis J. Immunopathology of the Lambert–Eaton myasthenic syndrome. *Springer Semin Immunopathol* 1995;17:3–15.

Le van Kim C, Mouro I, Cherif-Zahar B, et al. Molecular cloning and primary structure of the human blood group RhD polypeptide. *Proc Natl Acad Sci USA* 1992;89:10925–10929.

Lindstrom J. Immunobiology of myasthenia gravis, experimental autoimmune myasthenia gravis and Lambert–Eaton syndrome. Annu Rev Immunol 1985;3:109–131.

Mauro I, Colin Y, Chenif-Zahar B, et al. Molecular genetic basis of the human Rhesus blood group system. *Nature Genet* 1993;5:62–65.

Naparstek Y, Plotz PH. The role of autoantibodies in autoimmune disease. *Annu Rev Immunol* 1993;11:79–104.

Pichler WJ. Drug hypersensitivity reactions: classification and relationship to T-cell activation. In *Drug hypersensitivity 2007* (pp. 168-189). Karger Publishers.

Race R, Sanger R. *Blood groups in man.* 6th edn. Oxford: Blackwell Scientific Publications; 1975.

Rajan TV. The Gell–Coombs classification of hypersensitivity reactions: a re-interpretation. *TRENDS in Immunology.* 2003 Jul 1;24(7):376-9.

Riedl MA, Casillas AM. Adverse drug reactions: types and treatment options. *American family physician. 2003* Nov;68(9):1781-90.

Roitt's Essential Immunology, Peter J. Delves, Seamus J. Martin, Dennis R. Burton, Ivan M. Roitt. Thirteenth edition. Wiley-Blackwell.

Russo D, Redman C, Lee S. Association of XK and Kell blood group proteins. *J Biol Chem* 1998;273:13950–13956.

Schulz DR, Tozman EC. Anti-neutrophil cytoplasmic antibodies: major autoantigens, pathophysiology, and disease associations. *Semin Arthritis Rheum* 1995;25:143–159.

Uzzaman A, Cho SH. Classification of hypersensitivity reactions. *In Allergy & Asthma Proceedings* 2012 May 2 (Vol. 33).

Vincent A. Antibody-mediated disorders of neuro-muscular transmission. *Clin Neurophysiol Suppl* 2004;57:147–158.

Yamamoto F-I, Clausen H, White T, et al. Molecular genetic basis of the histo-blood group ABO system. *Nature* 1990;345:229.

In: The Fundamentals of Hypersensitivities … ISBN: 978-1-53617-012-2
Editor: Manzoor Ahmad Mir

Chapter 5

TYPE III HYPERSENSITIVITY (IMMUNE-COMPLEX MEDIATED HYPERSENSITIVITY)

Nissar A. Wani, Manzoor Ahmad Mir*, Umar Mehraj, Hina Qayoom, Safura Nisar, Bashir A. Sheikh and Syed Suhail

Department of Bioresources, School of Biological Sciences, University of Kashmir, Srinagar J&K, India

ABSTRACT

The Immune complexes are formed every time antibody meets antigen and are removed by the mononuclear phagocyte system following complement activation. Persistence of antigen from continued infection or in autoimmune disease can lead to immune complex disease. Immune complexes can trigger a variety of inflammatory processes. Immune complexes are normally removed by the mononuclear phagocyte system. Complement helps to disrupt antigen–antibody bonds and keeps immune complexes soluble. Primate erythrocytes bear a receptor for C3b and are

* Corresponding Author's Email: drmanzoor@kashmiruniversity.ac.in.

important for transporting complement containing immune complexes to the spleen for removal. Complement deficiencies lead to the formation of large, relatively insoluble complexes, which deposit in tissues. The size of immune complexes affects their deposition. Deposition of circulating, soluble immune complexes is limited by physical factors, such as the size and charge of the complexes. Small, positively charged complexes have the greatest propensity for deposition within vessels. Large immune complexes are rapidly removed in the liver and spleen. Immune complex deposition in the tissues results in tissue damage. Immune complexes can form both in the circulation, leading to systemic disease, and at local sites such as the lung. Charged cationic antigens have tissue-binding properties, particularly for the glomerulus, and help to localize complexes to the kidney. Factors that tend to increase blood vessel permeability enhance the deposition of immune complexes in tissues.

Keywords: immune-complex, C3b, C3a, C5a autoimmune disease, inhaled antigen, serum sickness, rheumatid arthritis, SLE, arthus reaction

OBJECTIVES

- Discuss the overall concept of Type III hypersensitivity reaction
- Describe how immune complexes can trigger a variety of inflammation processes
- Discuss the localized reaction of type III hypersensitivity
- Understand the generalized reaction of type III hypersensitivity
- Discuss the course of type III reaction
- Discuss various examples of Type III reaction

INTRODUCTION

Type III hypersensitivity is also called as Immune complex mediated hypersensitivity. The circulating immune complexes may lodge at various tissue sites where they activate complement and subsequently cause tissue cell lysis. Normally these complexes are phagocytosed effectively by the fixed monocytes and macrophages of the monocyte-macrophage system. In the presence of excess amounts of some soluble antigens, the antigen-antibody complexes may not be efficiently removed. Their accumulation can lead to a hypersensitivity reaction from complement that triggers a variety of inflammatory process. This form of hypersensitivity has a lot in common with type I except that the antibody involved is Ig G and therefore, not pre-bound to mast cells.

This reaction is mediated by immune antigen antibody complexes which promote tissue damage primarily through complement activation. Hypersensitivity type III reactions involve the interaction of immunoglobulin G with antigens to form immune complexes. It in turn triggers classical complement activation, leading to overproduction of other inflammatory mediators, leading to recruitment, activation and degranulation of peripheral blood granulocytes such as basophils or an influx of marginating neutrophils to specific tissues such as kidneys, lungs and joints culminating the damage.

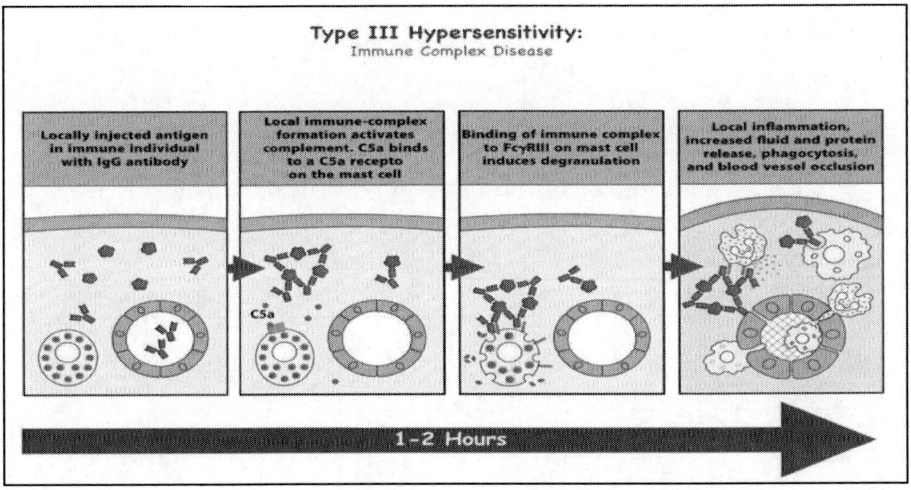

Figure 5.1. Representing the overview mechanism of type III hypersensitivity reaction.

Every time antigen enters the body, immune complexes are formed by the antibody and hence are eradicated effectively by the mononuclear phagocyte system. Occasionally, however, immune complexes persist and eventually deposit in a range of tissues and organs. The complement and effector cell-mediated damage that follows is known as a type III hypersensitivity reaction or immune complex disease. The magnitude of the reaction depends on the quantity of immune complexes as well as their distribution within the body.

The sites of immune complex deposition are partly determined by the localization of the antigen in the tissues and partly by how circulating complexes become deposited. Complex deposition, in particular, is frequently seen on blood-vessel walls, in the synovial membrane of joints, on the choroid plexus of brain and on the glomerular basement of kidney (Figure 5.1). This deposition of complexes initiates a reaction that results in the recruitment of neutrophils to the site. As a consequence, of granular release from the neutrophil, the tissue there is injured. The diseases resulting from immune complex formation can be broadly divided into three categories (Table 5.1)

- caused by inhalation of antigenic material
- due to autoimmune disease; and
- due to persistent infection

Table 5.1. Table indicating three categories of immune complex disease and source of the antigen and the organs most frequently affected

Cause	Antigen	Site of Complex Deposition
Persistent infection	**Microbial antigen**	**Infected organ(s)**
Autoimmunity	**Self-antigen**	**Kidney, joint, arteries, skin**
Inhaled antigen	**Mold, plant or animal antigen**	**Lung**

Immune Complexes Can Trigger a Variety of Inflammatory Processes

The immune complexes are also capable of generating a wide variety of inflammatory processes:

- they interact directly with basophils and platelets (via; Fc receptors) to induce the release of vasoactive amines (Figure 5.2);
- macrophages are stimulated to release cytokines, particularly tumor necrosis factor-α (TNFα) and interleukin-1 (IL-1), which have important roles in inflammation;
- they interact with the complement system to generate **C3a and C5a (anaphylatoxins)** – these complement fragments stimulate the release of vasoactive amines (including histamine and 5-hydroxytryptamine) and chemotactic factors from mast cells and basophils; and C5a is also chemotactic for basophils, eosinophils, and neutrophils.

Type III hypersensitive reactions develop when immune complexes activate the compliment system's array of effector molecules. The anaphylatoxin compliment split products, C3a, C4a and C5a cause endothelial cell retraction, localized mast-cell degranulation and consequent increase in local vascular permeability by the release of vasoactive amines by platelets, basophils, and mast, allowing the deposition of immune complexes on the blood vessel wall (Figure 5.2).

The deposited complexes continue to generate C3a and C5a. Platelets also aggregate on the exposed collagen of the vessel basement membrane to form microthrombi. The aggregated platelets continue to produce vasoactive amines and to stimulate the production of C3a and C5a. (Platelets are also a rich source of growth factors – these may be involved in the cellular proliferation seen in immune complex diseases such as glomerulonephritis and rheumatoid arthritis.)

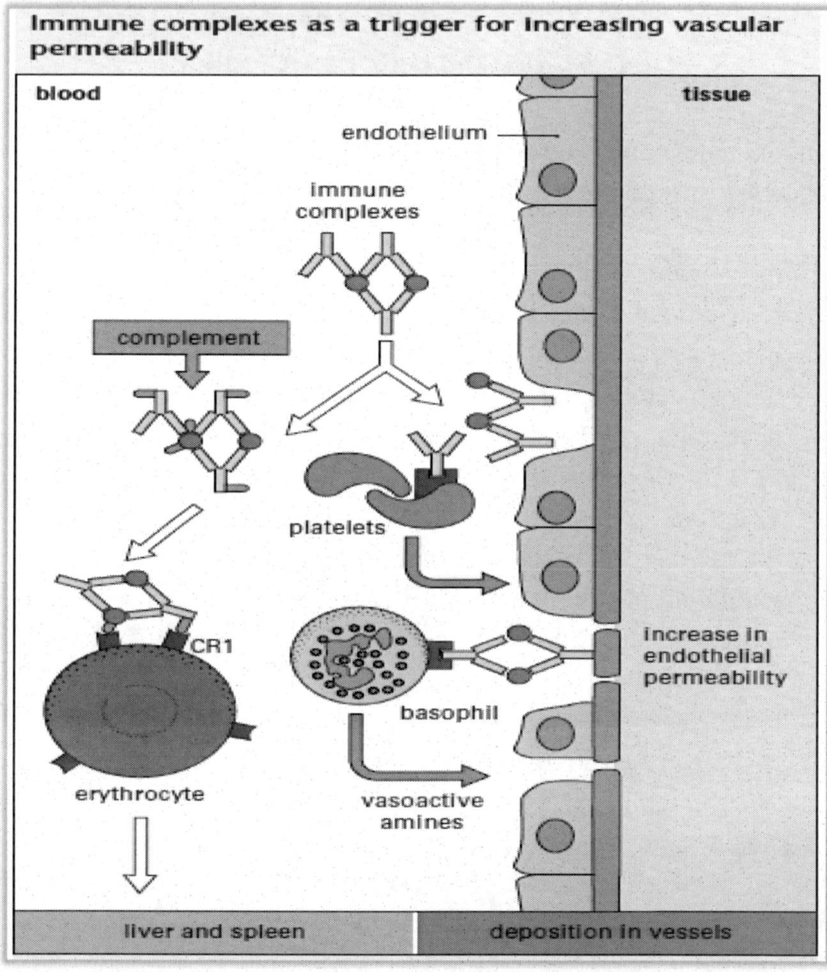

Figure 5.2. Immune complexes normally bind complement and are removed to the liver and spleen after binding to CR1 on erythrocytes. In inflammation, immune complexes act on basophils and platelets (in humans) to produce vasoactive amine release. The amines released (e.g., histamine, 5-hydroxytryptamine) cause endothelial cell retraction and thus increase vascular permeability.

Polymorphs are chemotactically attracted to the site by C5a. They attempt to engulf the deposited immune complexes, but are unable to do so because the complexes are bound to the vessel wall. They therefore exocytose their lysosomal enzymes onto the site of deposition (Figure 5.3).

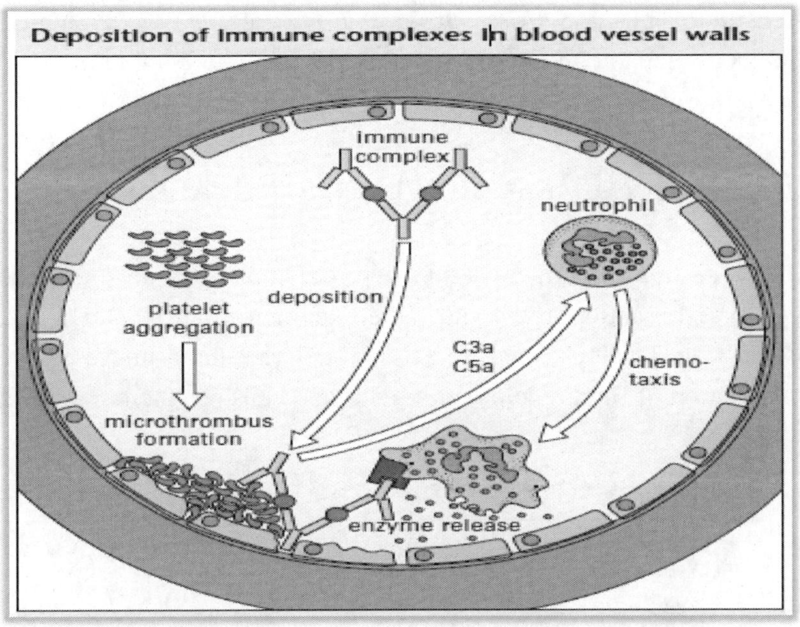

Figure 5.3. Increased vascular permeability allows immune complexes to be deposited in the blood vessel wall. This induces platelet aggregation and complement activation. The aggregated platelets form microthrombi on the exposed collagen of the basement membrane of the endothelium. Neutrophils are attracted to the site by complement products, but cannot ingest the complexes. They therefore exocytose their lysosomal enzymes, causing further damage to the vessel wall.

If simply released into the blood or tissue fluids these lysosomal enzymes are unlikely to cause much inflammation, because they are rapidly neutralized by serum enzyme inhibitors. But if the phagocyte applies itself closely to the tissue-trapped complexes through Fc binding, then serum inhibitors are excluded and the enzymes may damage the underlying tissue. The C3a, C5a and C5b67 are also chemotactic factors for neutrophils which can accumulate in large numbers at the site of immune-complex deposition. The larger immune-complexes are deposited on the basement membrane of blood-vessel walls or kidney glomerule, whereas smaller complexes may pass through the basement membrane and gets deposited in the sub-epithelium. Most of the tissue damage in type III hypersensitivity reaction arises from the release of lytic enzymes by neutrophils as they attempt to phagocytose the immune-complex.

TYPE III REACTION CAN BE LOCALIZED

After ingestion of antigen, a sensitive individual may develop a rapid, localized type I reaction at the site. Often, some 4-8 hours later, a typical Arthus reaction develops, localized tissue and vascular damage results in an accumulation of fluid (edema) and red blood cells (erythema) at the site.

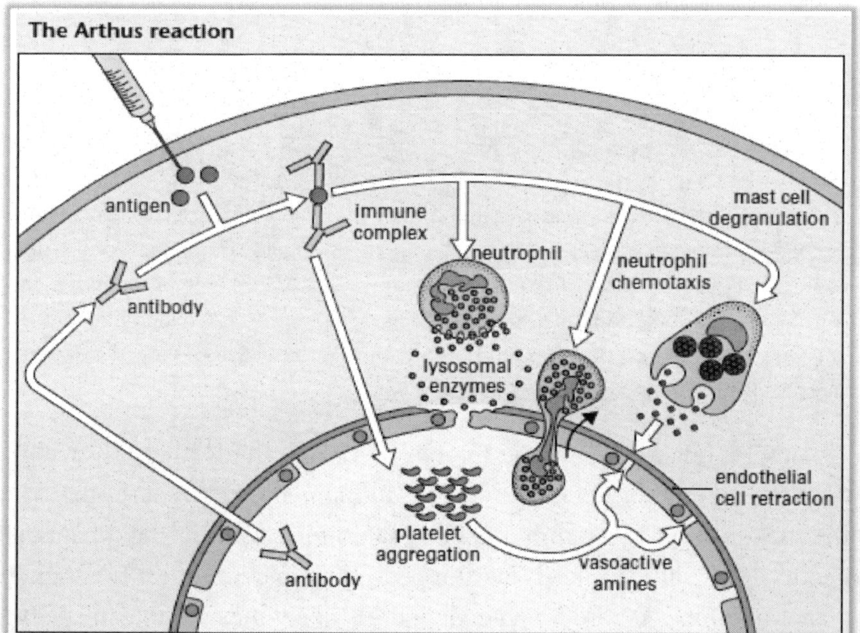

Figure 5.4. Antigen injected intradermally combines with specific antibody from the blood to form immune complexes. The complexes act on platelets and mast cells, which release vasoactive amines. Immune complexes also induce macrophages to release TNF and IL-1 (not shown). Mast cell products, including histamine and leukotrienes, induce increased blood flow and capillary permeability. The inflammatory reaction is potentiated by lysosomal enzymes released from the polymorphs. The Arthus reaction can be seen in patients with precipitating antibodies, such as those with extrinsic allergic alveolitis associated with farmer's lung disease.

The severity of the reaction can vary from mild swelling and redness to tissue necrosis. Intrapulmonary Arthus-type reaction induced by bacterial, spores, fungi or dried fecal protein can also cause pneumonitis or alveolitis. These reactions are known by a variety of common names reflecting the source of the antigen. This is exemplified in: "Farmer's lung" where there are circulating antibodies to thermophilic actinomycetes from moldy hay, and "pigeon fancier's disease" results from inhalation of a serum protein in dust derived from dried pigeon feces.

Both diseases are forms of **extrinsic allergic alveolitis**, and occur only after repeated exposure to the antigen. Note that the antibodies induced by these antigens are primarily IgG, rather than the IgE seen in type I hypersensitivity reactions. Again when the antigen enters the body by inhalation, local immune complexes are formed in the alveoli leading to inflammation and fibrosis (Figure 5.4).

Precipitating antibodies to actinomycete antigens are found in the sera of 90% of patients with farmer's lung. However, they are also found in some people with no disease, and are absent from some patients, so it seems that other factors are also involved in the disease process, including type IV hypersensitivity reactions.

Type III Hypersensitivity Reaction Can Also be Generalised

On exposure to large amounts of antigen, the antibody in the blood stream binds to these antigens, forming circulating immune complexes. Small complexes form if the antigens are in excess because these are not cleared easily by the phagocytic cells, and this can cause tissue-damaging type III reaction at various sites. Previously, generalized type III hypersensitivity reactions were often observed after the administration of antitoxins containing foreign serum, such as horse anti-tetanus or anti-diptheria serum. The recipient in such cases, develops specific antibodies for the foreign serum proteins forming circulating immune-complexes with the foreign serum epitopes (antigens). After exposure to foreign serum antigens, within weeks or days, an individual begins to develop a combination of symptoms that are called, **"Serum sickness"**. The symptoms include: generalized vasculitis (rashes) with edema and erythema, fever, arthritis and sometimes glomerulonephritis. This manifestation of serum sickness depend on the quantity of immune complexes formed as well as the overall size of the complexes, that determines the site of their deposition. The site of deposition may vary but generally these complexes accumulate in tissues where plasma's filtration occurs. From this, it is understood that serum sickness is the cause of high incidence of glomerulonephritis (complex deposition in the kidney) and arthritis (deposition in the synovial joints) and vasculitis (deposition in the arteries). Other than, serum sickness the formation of circulating immune complexes contributes to the pathogenesis of a number of conditions. It includes the following:

- Autoimmune Diseases- Systemic lupus erythematosus, Rheumatoid arthritis and Goodpasture's syndrome
- Drug Reactions- Allergies to penicillin and sulfonamides
- Infectious Diseases- Poststreptococcal glomerulonephritis, Meningitis, Hepatitis, Mononucleosis, Malaria, Trypanosomiasis

Complexes of antibody with various bacterial, viral, and parasitic antigens have been shown to induce a variety of type III hypersensitive reactions, including skin rashes, arthritic symptoms, and glomerulonephritis. Poststreptococcal glomerulonephritis, for example, develops when circulating complexes of antibody and streptococcal antigens are deposited in the kidney and damage the glomeruli. A number of autoimmune diseases stem from circulating complexes of antibody with self-proteins, with glycoproteins, or even with DNA. In systemic lupus erythematosus, complexes of DNA and anti-DNA antibodies accumulate in synovial membranes, causing arthritic symptoms, or accumulate on the basement membrane of the kidney, causing progressive kidney damage

Immune complex disease is a frequent complication of autoimmune disease. Immune complex disease is common in autoimmune disease, where the continued production of autoantibody to a self-antigen leads to prolonged immune complex formation. As the number of complexes in the blood increases, the systems responsible for the removal of complexes (mononuclear phagocyte, erythrocyte, and complement) become overloaded, and complexes are deposited in the tissues. Diseases with this etiology include:

- rheumatoid arthritis;
- systemic lupus erythematosus (SLE); and
- polymyositis.

Immune Complexes are Normally Removed by the Mononuclear Phagocyte System

Immune complexes are opsonized with C3b following complement activation, and removed by the mononuclear phagocyte system, particularly in the liver and spleen. Removal is mediated by the complement C3b receptor, CR1. In normal primates the erythrocytes provide a buffer mechanism, binding complexes that have fixed complement and effectively removing them from the plasma. In small blood vessels 'streamline flow' allows the erythrocytes to travel in the center of the vessel surrounded by the flowing plasma. Thus it is only the plasma that makes contact with the vessel wall. Only in the sinusoids of the liver and spleen, or at sites of turbulence, do the erythrocytes make contact with the lining of the vessels.

The complexes are transported to the liver and spleen, where they are removed by fixed tissue macrophages. Most of the CR1 is also removed in the process, so in situations of continuous immune complex formation the number of active receptors falls rapidly, impairing the efficiency of immune complex handling. In patients with SLE, for example, the number of receptors may well be halved. With fewer complement receptors the complexes are cleared rapidly to the liver, but these complexes, which arrive directly rather than on red cells, are later released into the circulation again and may then deposit in the tissues elsewhere and lead to inflammation. Complexes can also be released from erythrocytes in the circulation by the enzymatic action of factor I. This action leaves a small fragment (C3dg) attached to the CR1 on the cell membrane. These soluble complexes are then removed by phagocytic cells, particularly those in the liver, bearing receptors for IgG Fc

Complement Deficiency Impairs Clearance of Complexes

In patients with low levels of classical pathway components there is poor binding of immune complexes to erythrocytes. The complement deficiency may result from:

- depletion, caused by immune complex disease; or
- a hereditary disorder, as is the case in C2 deficiency

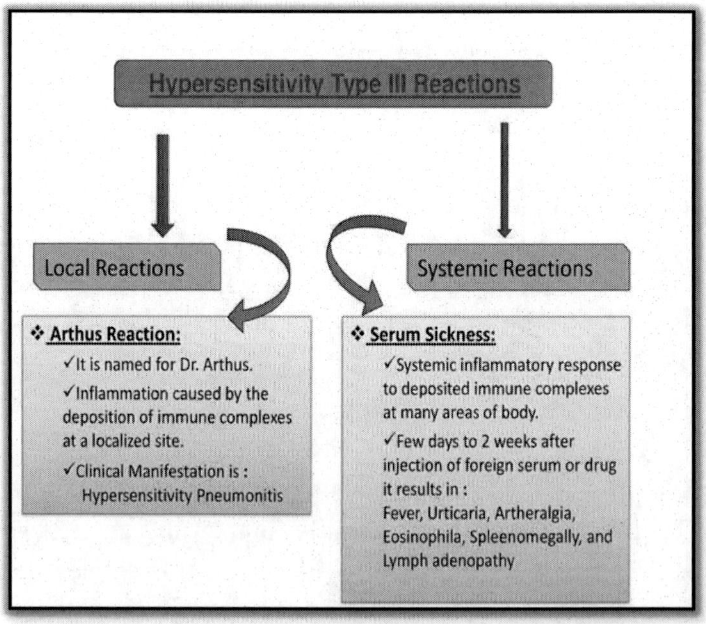

Figure 5.5. Showing two types of type III hypersensitivity reaction.

This might be expected to result in persistent immune complexes in the circulation, but in fact the reverse occurs, with the complexes disappearing rapidly from the circulation. These non-erythrocyte-bound complexes are taken up rapidly by the liver (but not the spleen) and are then released to be deposited in tissues such as skin, kidney, and muscle, where they can set up inflammatory reactions. Infusion of fresh plasma, containing complement, restores the clearance patterns to normal, illustrating the importance of complement in the clearance of immune complexes. Failure to localize in the spleen not only results in immune complex disease, but may also have important implications for the development of appropriate immune responses. This is because the spleen plays a vital role in antigen processing and the induction of immune responses

The Size of Immune Complexes Affects Their Deposition

In general, larger immune complexes are rapidly removed by the liver within a few minutes, whereas smaller complexes circulate for longer periods. This is because larger complexes are:

- more effective at binding to Fc receptors and at fixing complement, so binding better to erythrocytes;
- released more slowly from the erythrocytes by the action of factor I.

Anything that affects the size of complexes is therefore likely to influence clearance. It has been suggested that a genetic defect that favors the production of low-affinity antibody could lead to the formation of smaller complexes, and so to immune complex disease.

Antibodies to self-antigens may have low affinity and recognize only a few epitopes. This results in small complexes and long clearance times because the formation of large, cross-linked lattices is restricted. Affinity maturation is dependent on efficient somatic mutation and selection of B cells within germinal centers following binding of antigen. This process is far more effective when B cells are stimulated by antigen or immune complexes coated with complement. Patients with complement deficiencies are particularly prone to develop immune complex disease and recent evidence indicates that another way that this is brought about is through poor targeting of antigen complexes to germinal centers, so preventing affinity maturation.

Immune Complex Deposition in Tissues Results in Tissue Damage

Immune complexes may persist in the circulation for prolonged periods of time. However, simple persistence is not usually harmful in itself; the problems start only when complexes are deposited in the tissues.

Course of Hypersensitivity Type III Reaction

The formation of antigen antibody complexes occurs as a normal part on adaptive immune response. It is usually followed by Fc-receptor mediated recognition of the complexes by the phagocytes which engulf and destroy them and/or by complement activation resulting in the lysis of the cells on which the immune complexes are found. However, under certain conditions, immune complexes are inefficiently cleared and may be deposited in the blood vessels or tissues setting the stage for type III hypersensitivity response. These conditions include

- Presence of antigens capable of generating particularly extensive antigen – antibody lattices.
- A high intrinsic affinity of antigens for a particular tissue.
- The presence of highly charged antigens which can affect immune complex engulfment, and

- A compromised phagocytic system.

All these have been associated with the initiation of a type III response.

Examples of Hypersensitivity Type III Reaction

Autoimmune Diseases

Systemic lupus erythematosus: persistent antibody response to autoantigens is the characteristic feature of this disease. The complexes are deposited on the joints, kidneys and the skin of the patients. In SLE, autoantibodies are generated against cell contents including DNA, cytoplasmic proteins, and mitochondria.

Immune complexes form whenever cell contents are released and these deposit in capillary beds in organs such as skin, kidney, joint, and brain where they activate complement causing further tissue damage. Here complement is playing dual roles:

- The important immune complex solubilizing roles will prevent immune complex deposition until the capacity of the system is exceeded;
- Beyond this threshold complexes deposit and activate complement in the tissues, causing pathology.

Patients with SLE often have both systemic (multiorgan) and localised manifestations. Complement changes from hero to villain. Patients with SLE often have markedly decreased plasma levels of complement activity and the components C3 and C4 due to the massive and widespread activation of the system. Levels of these parameters can be used to monitor disease activity

Rheumatoid arthritis (RA) it is a chronic inflammatory disease that mainly affects the joints. Rheumatoid factor, an IgM autoantibody is found in serum and synovial fluid of most RA patients. It binds to the Fc region of normal IgG. These immune complexes result in inflammation of joints.

Infectious Diseases

Poststreptococcal glomerulonephritis: It is a disorder of kidneys that occurs after infection with certain strains of streptococcus bacteria. The infection itself does not occur in the kidneys, but in different parts like skin and throat. The bacterial infection causes the inflammation of glomeruli.

CONCLUSION

A type III hypersensitive reaction is mediated by the formation of immune complexes and the ensuing activation of complement. Complement split products serve as immune effector molecules that elicit localized vasodilation and chemotactically attract neutrophils. Deposition of immune complexes near the site of antigen entry can induce an Arthus reaction, in which lytic enzymes released by the accumulated neutrophils and the complement membrane attack complex cause localized tissue damage.

MULTIPLE CHOICE QUESTIONS (MCQS)

1. **Which of the following hypersensitivities are immune complex mediated?**
   A. Type I hypersensitivity
   B. Type II hypersensitivity
   C. Type III hypersensitivity
   D. Type IV hypersensitivity

2. **Which of the following are examples of type III hypersensitivity?**
   A. Multiple Sclerosis and Contact Dermatitis
   B. Rheumatoid Arthritis and Arthus reaction
   C. Allergies and Asthma
   D. Myasthenia Gravis and Graves' Disease

3. **Immune complex disease**
   A. requires cytotoxic T cells.
   B. requires neutrophils
   C. usually involves IgE.
   D. usually involves IgA.

4. **Serum sickness occurs only**
   A. when anti-basement-membrane antibodies are present.
   B. in cases of extreme excess of antibody.
   C. when IgE antibody is produced.
   D. when soluble immune complexes are formed.
   E. in the absence of neutrophils.

5. **Both immune complex disease and delayed type hypersensitivity involve**
   A. phagocytic cells.
   B. IgG or IgM antibodies.
   C. NK lymphocytes.
   D. B cells.

6. **The broad spectrum of autoantibody formation in patients with systemic lupus erythematosus is probably indicative of**
   A. excess production of macrophages.
   B. failed regulation of a multi-specific B-cell clone.
   C. the presence of many auto-reactive B-cell clones.
   D. heterozygosity at the HLA B locus.

7. Complement receptors on red blood cells and Fc receptors on platelets probably facilitate

A. immune phagocytosis of immune complexes by RBCs & platelets.
B. immune pinocytosis of immune complexes by RBCs & platelets.
C. the synthesis of gamma interferon by the platelet.
D. the elimination of immune complexes by phagocytic cells.

8. Rheumatoid arthritis is an ____ disease that affects the ____

A. Allergic/cartilage
B. Autoimmune/nerves
C. Autoimmune/joints
D. Immunodeficiency/muscles
E. Allergic/muscles

9. An example of a type III immune complex disease is:

A. Contact dermatitis
B. Graft rejection
C. Serum sickness
D. Atopy
E. Allergies

10. Which of the following is considered an autoimmune disease?

A. Rheumatoid arthritis
B. AIDS
C. SCID
D. Agammaglobulinemia

11. A condition in which individual fails to recognize its own parts as self and develops an immune response against its own cells and tissues is called:

A. Phagocytosis
B. Inflammation
C. Necrosis
D. Autoimmunity

12. Phagocytosis

A. is carried by cells of the adaptive immune system.
B. is restricted to macrophages.
C. is important in bacterial infections.
D. is a process that does not involve energy.
E. results in division of the cell.

13. Inflammation resulting from IgG–antigen complexes

A. requires IgM to activate complement.
B. involves complement activation.
C. produces the rash of poison ivy.
D. requires T cells.

14. Which of the following is a known inhibitor of inflammation

A. TNFα.
B. nerve growth factor.
C. protein C.
D. neuropeptide Y.
E. reactive oxygen species.

15. Direct causes of inflammation include

A. TGFβ.
B. histaminase.
C. ICAM-1.
D. VCAM.
E. LPS.

ANSWER KEY:

1.C, 2.B, 3.B, 4.D, 5.A, 6.C, 7.D, 8.C, 9.C, 10.A, 11.D, 12.C, 13.B, 14.C, 15.E

FREQUENTLY ASKED QUESTIONS (FAQS)

1. Define immune complex mediated (type III) hypersensitivity?

Answer: This type of hypersensitivity is also called as Immune complex mediated hypersensitivity. This reaction is mediated by immune antigen antibody complexes which promote tissue damage primarily through complement activation. Hypersensitivity type III reactions involve the interaction of immunoglobulin G or immunoglobulin M with antigens to form immune complexes. It in turn triggers classical complement activation, leading to overproduction of other inflammatory mediators, leading to recruitment, activation and degranulation of peripheral blood granulocytes such as basophils or an influx of marginating neutrophils to specific tissues such as kidneys, lungs and joints culminating the damage.

2. Outline the two types of hypersensitivity type III reaction?

Answer: The two types of hypersensitivity type III reaction are:

- Localized Type III hypersensitivity reaction (Arthus reaction): When antigen is injected or enters intradermally or subcutaneously, they bind with antibody to form localized immune complexes which mediate acute Arthus reaction within 4 to 8 hours.
- Generalized Type III hypersensitivity reaction: When large amount of antigen enters blood stream and bind to antibody, circulating immune complexes forms. If antigens are in significantly excess compared to antibody, the immune complexes formed are smaller and soluble which are not phagocytosed by phagocytic cells leading to Type III hypersensitivity reaction.

3. What are immune complexes?

Answer: Immune complex is the term used to refer to the combination of an antibody with its antigen. Immune complexes must be removed from tissues and kept from accumulating in the circulation and forming deposits throughout the body. Failure to clear immune complexes can lead to autoimmune disease.

4. Explain how immune complexes trigger inflammation.

Answer: The immune complexes are also capable of generating a wide variety of inflammatory processes:

- they interact directly with basophils and platelets (via; Fc receptors) to induce the release of vasoactive amines (Figure 5.2);
- macrophages are stimulated to release cytokines, particularly tumor necrosis factor-α (TNFα) and interleukin-1 (IL-1), which have important roles in inflammation;
- they interact with the complement system to generate **C3a and C5a (anaphylatoxins)** – these complement fragments stimulate the release of vasoactive amines (including histamine and 5-hydroxytryptamine) and chemotactic factors from mast cells and basophils; and C5a is also chemotactic for basophils, eosinophils, and neutrophils.

Type III hypersensitive reactions develop when immune complexes activate the compliment system's array of effector molecules. The anaphylatoxin compliment split products, C3a, C4a and C5a cause endothelial cell retraction, localized mast-cell degranulation and consequent increase in local vascular permeability by the release of vasoactive amines by platelets, basophils, and mast, allowing the deposition of immune complexes on the blood vessel wall. The deposited complexes continue to generate C3a and C5a.

5. What is Arthus reaction?

Answer: Arthus reaction is a type of hypersensitivity reaction produced by local formation of antigen-antibody aggregates that activate the complement cascade and hence cause thrombosis, haemorrhage and acute inflammation.

6. Name the diseases resulting from immune complex formation.

Answer: The disease caused by the formation of immune complex can be broadly divided into three categories.

- Inhalation of antigenic material
- Autoimmune disease; and
- Persistent infection

7. What do you mean by Complement deficiency impairs clearance of complexes?

Answer: In patients with low levels of classical pathway components there is poor binding of immune complexes to erythrocytes. The complement deficiency may result from:

- depletion, caused by immune complex disease; or
- a hereditary disorder, as is the case in C2 deficiency

This might be expected to result in persistent immune complexes in the circulation, but in fact the reverse occurs, with the complexes disappearing rapidly from the circulation. These non-erythrocyte-bound complexes are taken up rapidly by the liver (but not the spleen) and are then released to be deposited in tissues such as skin, kidney, and muscle, where they can set up inflammatory reactions. Infusion of fresh plasma, containing complement, restores the clearance patterns to normal, illustrating the importance of complement in the clearance of immune complexes. Failure to localize in the spleen not only results in immune complex disease, but may also have important implications for the development of appropriate immune responses.

8. What is serum sickness?

Answer: generalized type III hypersensitivity reactions were often observed after the administration of antitoxins containing foreign serum, such as horse anti-tetanus or anti-diptheria serum. The recipient in such cases, develops specific antibodies for the foreign serum proteins forming circulating immune-complexes with the foreign serum epitopes (antigens). After exposure to foreign serum antigens, within weeks or days, an individual begins to develop a combination of symptoms that are called, "Serum sickness".

9. Which antibody is involved in type III hypersensitivity reaction?

Answer: IgG antibody is involved in inducing the type III hypersensitivity reaction.

10. What is systemic lupus erythematosus (SLE)?

Answer: Persistent antibody response to autoantigens is the characteristic feature of this disease. The complexes are deposited on the joints, kidneys and the skin of the patients. In SLE, autoantibodies are generated against cell contents including DNA, cytoplasmic proteins, and mitochondria.

Immune complexes form whenever cell contents are released and these deposit in capillary beds in organs such as skin, kidney, joint, and brain where they activate complement causing further tissue damage. Here complement is playing dual roles:

- The important immune complex solubilizing roles will prevent immune complex deposition until the capacity of the system is exceeded;
- Beyond this threshold complexes deposit and activate complement in the tissues, causing pathology.

11. What is Rheumatid arthritis (RA)?

Answer: Rheumatoid arthritis (RA) is a chronic inflammatory disease that mainly affects the joints. Rheumatoid factor, an IgM autoantibody is found in serum and synovial fluid of most RA patients. It binds to the Fc region of normal IgG. These immune complexes result in inflammation of joints.

12. How size of immune complexes affects their deposition?

Answer: In general, larger immune complexes are rapidly removed by the liver within a few minutes, whereas smaller complexes circulate for longer periods. This is because larger complexes are:

- more effective at binding to Fc receptors and at fixing complement, so binding better to erythrocytes;
- released more slowly from the erythrocytes by the action of factor I.

Anything that affects the size of complexes is therefore likely to influence clearance.

13. The formation of circulating immune complexes results in.....

Answer: The formation of circulating immune complexes contributes to the pathogenesis of a number of conditions. It includes the following:

- Autoimmune Diseases- Systemic lupus erythematosus, Rheumatoid arthritis and Goodpasture's syndrome
- Drug Reactions- Allergies to penicillin and sulfonamides
- Infectious Diseases- Poststreptococcal glomerulonephritis, Meningitis, Hepatitis, Mononucleosis, Malaria, Trypanosomiasis

14. Explain localized type III reaction.

Answer: After ingestion of antigen, a sensitive individual may develop a rapid, localized type I reaction at the site. Often, some 4-8 hours later, a typical Arthus reaction develops, localized tissue and vascular damage results in an accumulation of fluid (edema) and red blood cells (erythema) at the site. The severity of the reaction can vary from mild swelling and redness to tissue necrosis.

15. What is farmer's lung disease and pigeon fancier's disease?

Answer: Intrapulmonary Arthus-type reaction induced by bacterial, spores, fungi or dried fecal protein can also cause pneumonitis or alveolitis. These reactions are known by a variety of common names reflecting the source of the antigen. This is exemplified in: "Farmer's lung" where there are circulating antibodies to thermophilic actinomycetes from moldy hay, and "pigeon fancier's disease" results from inhalation of a serum protein in dust derived from dried pigeon feces.

ASSIGNMENTS

Q1. Briefly describe the course, clinical findings, and mode of treatment of immune-complex mediated hypersensitivity?

Q2. Discuss the various possible underlying causes of type III hypersensitivity reaction?

Q3. What do you understand by Arthus reaction?

Q4. Define hypersensitivity type III, illustrating the initiating cells and molecules that bring about the pathological effects.

Q5. Explain the two types of type III hypersensitivity with examples.

Q6. Describe serum sickness. Give suitable examples

REFERENCES

Arthus, M. Injections répétées de sérum de cheval chez le lapin [Repeated injections of horse serum in rabbits]. *C R Seances Soc Biol Filiales*, 1903, 55, 817.

Birmingham, DJ; Herbert, LA; Cosio, FG; et al. Immune complex erythrocyte complement receptor interactions *in vivo* during induction of glomerulonephritis in non-human primates. *J Lab Clin Med*, 1990, 116, 242–252.

Boackle, SA; Holer, VM; Karp, DR. CD21 augments antigen presentation in immune individuals. *Eur J Immunol*, 1997, 27, 122–129.

Boruchov, AM; Heller, G; Veri, MC; et al. Activating and inhibitory IgG Fc receptors on human DCs mediate opposing functions. *J Clin Invest*, 2005, 115, 2914–2923.

Bruhns, P; Samuelsson, A; Pollard, JW; Ravetch, JV. Colony-stimulating factor-1-dependent macrophages are responsible for IVIG protection in antibody-induced autoimmune disease. *Immunity*, 2003, 18, 573–581.

Clynes, R; Maizes, JS; Guinamard, R; et al. Modulation of immune complex-induced inflammation *in vivo* by the co-ordinate expression of activation and inhibitory Fc receptors. *J Exp Med*, 1999, 189, 179–185.

Cornacoff, JB; Hebert, LA; Smead, WL; et al. Primate erythrocyte immune complex clearing mechanism. *J Clin Invest*, 1983, 71, 236– 247.

Davies, KA; Schifferli, JA; Walport, MJ. Complement deficiency and immune complex diseases. *Springer Semin Immunopathol*, 1994, 15, 397–416.

Dixon, FJ; Joseph, D; Feldman, JD; et al. Experimental glomerulonephritis: the pathogenesis of a laboratory model resembling the spectrum of human glomerulonephritis. *J Exp Med*, 1961, 113, 899–919.

Dixon, FJ; Vazquez, JJ; Weigle, WO; et al. Pathogenesis of serum sickness. *Arch Pathol*, 1958, 65, 18–28.

Emlen, W; Carl, V; Burdick, CG. Mechanism of transfer of immune complexes from red blood cell CR1 to monocytes. *Clin Exp Immunol*, 1992, 89, 8–17.

Finbloom, DS; Magilvary, DB; Harford, JB; et al. Influence of antigen on immune complex behaviour in mice. *J Clin Invest*, 1981, 68, 214–224.

Fukuyama, H; Nimmerjahn, F; Ravetch, JV. The inhibitory Fc gamma receptor modulates autoimmunity by limiting the accumulation of immunoglobulin G+ anti-DNA plasma cells. *Nat Immunol*, 2005, 6, 99–106.

Heidelberger, M. Quantitative chemical studies on complement or a lexin. *J Exp Med*, 1941, 73, 681–709.

Inman, RD. Immune complexes in SLE. *Clin Rheum Dis*, 1982, 8, 49–62.

Johnston, A; Auda, GR; Kerr, MA; et al. Dissociation of primary antigen–antibody bonds is essential for complement mediated solubilization of immune complexes. *Mol Immunol*, 1992, 29, 659–665.

Kijlstrea, H; Van Es, LA; Daha, MR. The role of complement in the binding and degradation of immunoglobulin aggregates by macrophages. *J Immunol*, 1979, 123, 2488–2493.

Lachmann, PJ. Complement deficiency and the pathogenesis of autoimmune complex disease. *Chem Immunol*, 1980, 49, 245–263.

Lucisano Valim, M; Lachmann, PJ. The effects of antibody isotype and antigenic epitope density on the complement-fixing activity of immune complexes: a systematic study using chimeric anti-NIP antibodies with human Fc regions. *Clin Exp Immunol*, 1991, 84, 1–8.macrophages.

McGaha, TL; Sorrentino, B; Ravetch, JV. Restoration of tolerance in lupus by targeted inhibitory receptor expression. *Science*, 2005, Jan 28, 307, 590–593.

McKenzie, SE; Taylor, SM; Malladi, P; et al. The role of the human Fc receptor FcγRIIA in the immune clearance of platelets: a transgene mouse model. *J Immunol*, 1999, 162, 4311–4318.

Miller, GW; Nussenzweig, V. A new complement function: solubilization of antigen–antibody aggregates. *Proc Natl Acad Sci*, 1975, 72, 418–422.

Moll, T; Nitschke, L; Carroll, M; et al. A critical role for Fc gamma RIIB in the induction of rheumatoid factors. *J Immuno ln*, 2004, 173, 4724–4728.

Olsson, M; Bruhns, P; Frazier, WA; et al. Platelet homeostasis is regulated by platelet expression of CD47 under normal conditions and in passive immune thrombocytopenia. *Blood*, 2005, 105, 3577–3582.

Park, SY; Ueda, S; Ohno, H; et al. Resistance of Fc receptor-deficient mice to fatal glomerulonephritis. *J Clin Invest*, 1998, 102, 1229–1238.

Qiao, JH; Castellani, LW; Fishbein, MC; et al. Immune complex mediated vasculitis increases coronary artery lipid accumulation in autoimmune-prone MRL mice. *Arterioscler Thromb*, 1993, 13, 932–943.

Ravetch, JV. A full complement of receptors in immune complex diseases. *J Clin Invest*, 2002, 110, 1759–1761.

Ravetch, JV. Fc receptors. *Curr Opin Immunol*, 1997, 9, 121–125.

Schifferli, JA; Ng, YC; Peters, DK. The role of complement and its receptor in the elimination of immune complexes. *N Engl J Med*, 1986, 315, 488–495.

Sylvestre, DL; Ravetch, JV. A dominant role for mast cell Fc receptors in the Arthus reaction. *Immunity*, 1996, 5, 387–390.

Takata, Y; Tamura, N; Fujita, T. Interaction of C3 with antigen–antibody complexes in the process of solubilisation of immune precipitates. *J Immunol*, 1984, 132, 2531–2537.

Terino, FL; Powell, MS; McKenzie, IF; Hogarth, PM. Recombinant soluble human FcγRII: production, characterization, and inhibition of the Arthus reaction. *J Exp Med*, 1993, 178, 1617– 1628.

The ofilopoulos, AN; Dixon, FJ. The biology and detection of immune complexes. *Adv Immunol*, 1979, 28, 89–220.

Warren, JS; Yabroff, KR; Remick, DG; et al. Tumour necrosis factor participates in the pathogenesis of acute immune complex alveolitis in the rat. *J Clin Invest*, 1989, 84, 1873–1882.

In: The Fundamentals of Hypersensitivities … ISBN: 978-1-53617-012-2
Editor: Manzoor Ahmad Mir

Chapter 6

TYPE IV HYPERSENSITIVITY (DELAYED TYPE HYPERSENSITIVITY)

Nissar A. Wani, Syed Suhail, Hina Qayoom, Safura Nisar, Bashir A. Sheikh, Umar Mehraj and Manzoor Ahmad Mir*

Department of Bioresources, School of Biological Sciences, University of Kashmir, Srinagar J&K, India

ABSTRACT

Type IV hypersensitivity (delayed type hypersensitivity) is cell mediated and not antibody mediated. It is the only class of hypersensitive reactions which are triggered by antigen-specific T-cells. This is mediated by T-cell dependent effector mechanism involving T_H cells, primarily of the T_H1 subtype, but in a few cases T_C-cells. Antibodies do not play a role in Type IV hypersensitivity reactions. The tuberculin skin test is an example of Type IV hypersensitivity. This test is done by putting a small amount of tuberculin purified protein derivative (PPD) under the top layer of skin. If any person has ever been exposed to the Mycobacterium tuberculosis, skin will react to the antigens by developing a firm red bump at the site within 2 days. It is a standard method of determining whether a person is infected with mycobacterium tuberculosis. Contact dermatitis is another example of Type IV hypersensitivity reaction. DTH responses are responsible for granulomas associated with tuberculosis. DTH requires T cells to be sensitized to the antigen. Subsequent re-exposure to antigen results in cytokine generation, inflammation and recruitment of macrophages. A Type IV hypersensitive reaction involves the cell-mediated branch of the immune system. Antigen activation of sensitized T_H1 cells induces release of various cytokines that cause macrophages to accumulate and become activated. The net effect of the activation of macrophages is to release lytic enzymes that cause localized tissue damage

Keywords: Type IV hypersensitivity reaction, T_H1 cells, cytokines, DTH, contact hypersensitivity, tuberculin type hypersensitivity, granulomatous hypersensitivity

OBJECTIVES

- Understand the concept of delayed type hypersensitivity
- To know about the historical perspective of DTH
- Describe the course of Type IV hypersensitivity
- Discuss the contact hypersensitivity
- Describe some of the clinical findings about Type IV reaction
- Discuss about diagnostics and treatment of DTH

INTRODUCTION

Type IV hypersensitivity reaction is commonly referred to as Delayed type hypersensitivity (DTH) and it is the only hypersensitivity category that is purely cell-mediated, rather than antibody mediated. Delayed type hypersensitivity is an injurious cytokine-mediated inflammatory reaction resulting from the activation of T cells. The reaction is called hypersensitivity because It reflects excessive i.e., injurious immune responses and delayed because it typically develops during 24 to 48 hours after antigen challenge. Whereas antibody can be present in a preformed state, antigen-specific T cells need time to proliferate and then synthesize and secrete cytokines – hence referred to as *"Delayed Type Hypersensitivity"* (Figure 6.1).

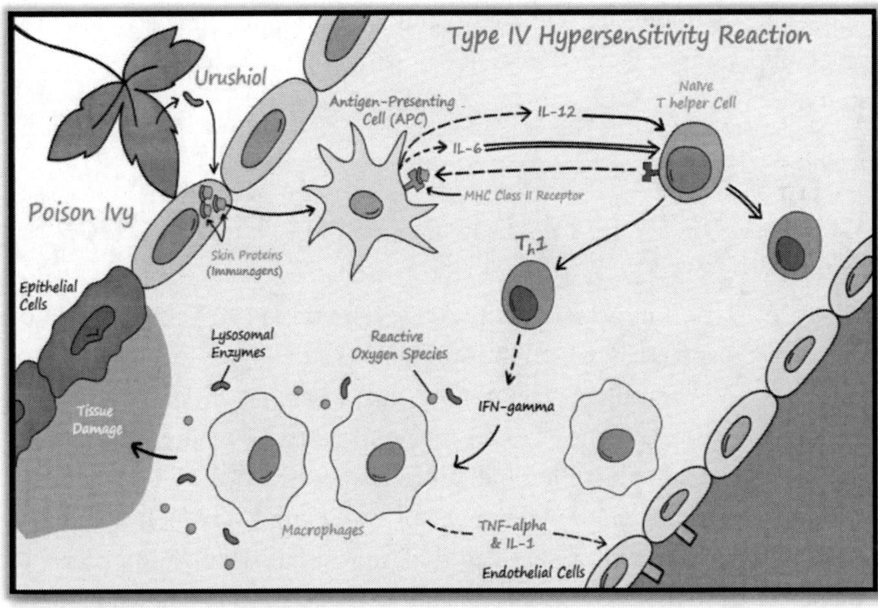

Figure 6.1. Showing the overall Type IV hypersensitivity reaction.

HISTORICAL PERSPECTIVE OF TYPE IV HYPERSENSITIVITY REACTION

Type IV reaction was described first by Robert Koch in 1890, he observed that the individuals infected with Mycobaterium tuberclosis, developed a localised inflammatory response when injected intradermally with a filtrate derived from a mycobacterial culture. He then called this localised skin reaction a, "tuberculin reaction". However, with time it became apparent that a variety of other antigenic epitopes could induce this response. In reference, to the delayed onset of the reaction and to the tissue damage (hypersensitivity) that is often associated with it, its name was changed to delayed-type or Type IV reaction.

The hall mark of a Type IV reaction is the delay in time that is required for the reaction to develop and the recruitment of macrophages as opposed to neutrophils as found in a Type III reaction. With macrophages being the major component of this reaction, which surrounds the site of inflammation.

Course of Type IV Hypersensitivity Reaction

Delayed type hypersensitivity (DTH) is a T cell mediated inflammatory response in which the stimulation of antigen specific effector T cell leads to macrophage activation and localized inflammation and edema within tissues. The T cell response may be directed against exogenous agents, such as microbial antigens and sensitizing chemicals or against self-antigens. The development of the Type IV response initiates after primary contact with an antigen with an initial sensitization phase of 1-2 weeks. During this period, T_H cells are activated and expanded clonally by antigen presenting class II MHC cells. Furthermore, a variety of cells have been shown to be involved in the activation of a DTH response, including Langerhans cells found in the epidermis. These cells take up the antigen which enters through the skin and transfer it to regional lymph nodes, where T cells are activated by the antigen. The T cells activated during this phase (sensitization) are $CD4^+$, typically of the sub-type T_H1, in some cases $CD8^+$ cells have also been shown to induce a DTH response. On subsequent exposure, the antigen induces the effector phase of the Type IV response (Figure 6.2). In this phase, the T_H1 cells secrete a variety of cytokines that recruit and also activate macrophages and also other non-specific inflammatory cells. Subsequent exposure of the sensitized individual to the antigen, either injected intradermally or applied to the epidermis, results in the recruitment of antigen-specific T cells to the site and the development of a local inflammatory response over 24–72 hours. Once a Type IV response initiates, a number of non-specific cells and active mediators are set in to play, resulting in their enhanced amplification. Macrophages are the main effector cells of this response, with only the 5% involvement of antigen-specific T_H1 cells. Cytokine release induce blood monocytes to stick to endothelial cells and migrate into the surrounding tissue from blood. It is during this process, the monocytes differentiate into activated macrophages (Figure 6.3). These activated macrophages show increased levels of phagocytic activity and heightened release of lytic enzymes in the area of infection leading to non-specific destruction of cells and hence of the intracellular pathogen. The influx and activation of macrophages in the Type IV response are important in host defense against parasites and bacteria that live within cells, where circulating antibodies cannot reach. If the foreign antigen persists in the tissues, chronic activation of T cells and macrophages may lead to granuloma formation and tissue damage. If the antigen is an organ-specific self-antigen, autoreactive T cells may produce localized cellular inflammation resulting in autoimmune disease, such as Type I diabetes mellitus.

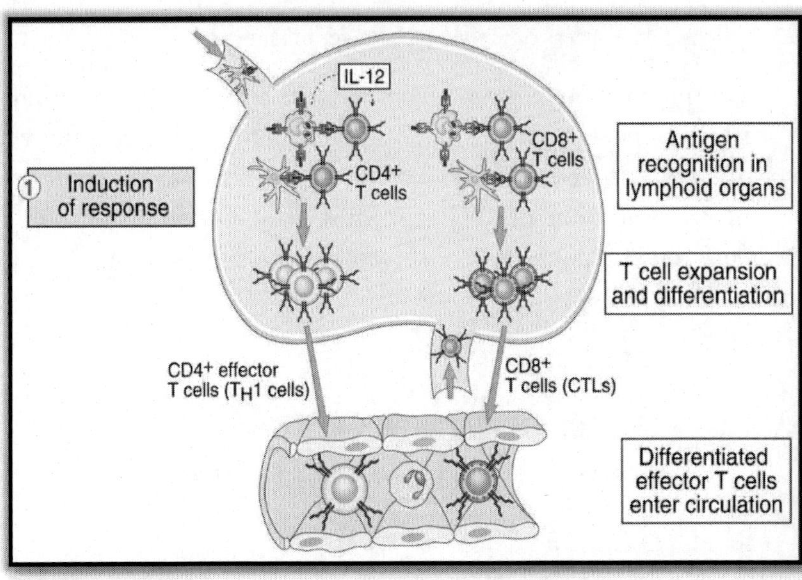

Figure 6.2. Represents the mechanism of delayed type hypersensitivity reaction.

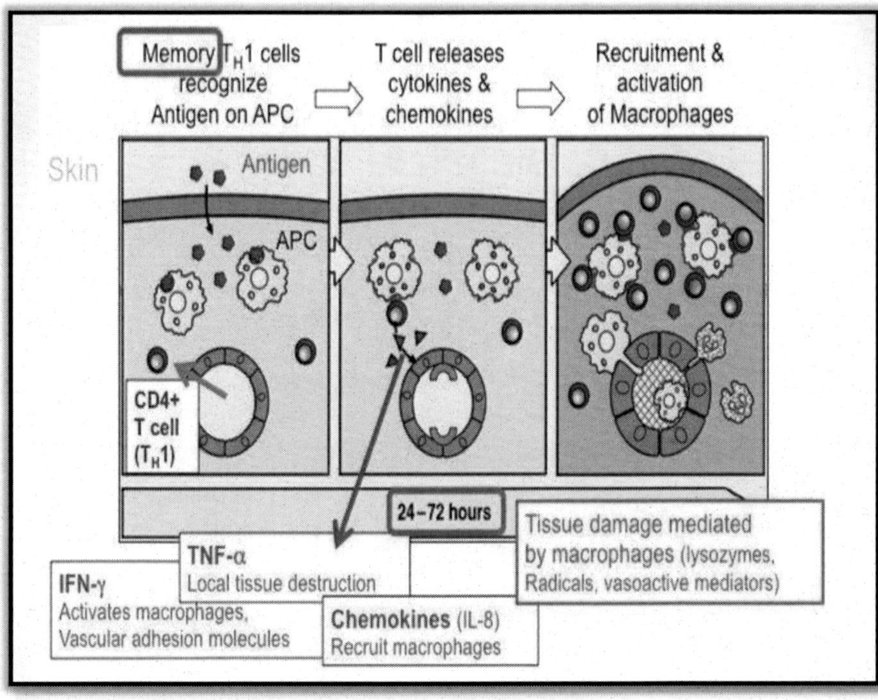

Figure 6.3. Showing the process of activation of macrophages.

When continuous activation of macrophages induces the macrophage to stick closely to one another, fusing to form a multi-nucleated giant cells. These cells displace the normal tissue cells, forming palpable nodules, and release high concentration of lytic enzymes which destroy surrounding tissue. In these situations, the response can destroy blood vessels and lead to extensive tissue necrosis.

Contact Hypersensitivity Occurs at the Point of Contact with an Allergen

Contact hypersensitivity is characterized by an eczematous reaction in the skin at the point of contact with an allergen (Figure 6.4.). It is often seen following contact with agents such as nickel, chromate, rubber accelerators, and pentadecacatechol, which is the sensitizing agent in poison ivy. This is distinct from the non-immune-mediated inflammatory response to irritants. The immunologically active components of sensitizing agents are called *haptens.* Haptens are:

- too small to be antigenic by themselves, having a molecular weight often less than 1 kDa;
- lipophilic and penetrate the epidermis where they conjugate, most often covalently, to self-proteins to form *neo-antigens.*

Type IV hypersensitivity reactions are mediated by antigen-specific effector T cells		
Syndrome	**Antigen**	**Consequence**
Delayed-type hypersensitivity	**Proteins:** **Insect venom** **Mycobacterial proteins (tuberculin, lepromin)**	**Local skin swelling:** **Erythema** **Induration** **Cellular infiltrate** **Dermatitis**
Contact hypersensitivity	**Haptens:** **Pentadecacatechol (poison ivy)** **DNFB** **Small metal ions:** **Nickel** **Chromate**	**Local epidermal reaction:** **Erythema** **Cellular infiltrate** **Vesicles** **Intraepidermal abscesses**
Gluten-sensitive enteropathy (celiac disease)	**Gliadin**	**Villous atrophy in small bowel** **Malabsorption**

Figure 6.4. Type-IV hypersensitivity reactions are mediated by antigen-specific effector T cells

The sensitizing potential of a hapten cannot reliably be predicted from its chemical structure, though there is some correlation with the ability of the molecule to penetrate the skin and the number of haptens attached to the carrier protein. Some potent haptens, such as dinitrochlorobenzene (DNCB), sensitize nearly all individuals and can be used to assess cell-mediated immunity. DNCB applied to the skin binds to epidermal proteins and to MHC-

Many contact-dermatitis reactions, including the responses to formaldehyde, trinitrophenol, nickel, turpentine, and active agents in various cosmetics and hair dyes, poison oak, and poison ivy, are mediated by TH1 cells. Most of these substances are small molecules that can complex with skin proteins. This complex is internalized by antigen-presenting cells in the skin (e.g., Langerhans cells), then processed and presented together with class II MHC molecules, causing activation of sensitized TH1 cells. In the reaction to poison oak, for example, a pentadecacatechol compound from the leaves of the plant forms a complex with skin proteins. When TH cells react with this compound appropriately displayed by local antigen-presenting cells, they differentiate into sensitized TH1 cells. A subsequent exposure to pentadecacatechol will elicit activation of TH1 cells and induce cytokine production. Approximately 48–72 h after the second exposure, the secreted cytokines cause macrophages to accumulate at the site. Activation of these macrophages and release of lytic enzymes result in the redness and pustules that characterize a reaction to poison oak.

Tuberculin-type hypersensitivity may also be induced by T cell responses to non-microbial antigens, such as beryllium and zirconium.

CLINICAL FINDINGS

Type IV reactions take days to weeks to manifest. Symptoms vary with the type and severity of the hypersensitivity reaction. Type IV hypersensitivity reaction can occur in many parts of the body. Generally they include skin, lungs, pancreas, thyroid etc. Itching and skin rash or utricaria (hives) are common with Type I hypersensitivity reaction. Type IV hypersensitivity is involved in the pathogenesis of many autoimmune and infectious diseases such as tuberculosis, leprosy, blastomycosis, histoplasmosis, toxoplasmosis, Leishmaniasis etc. and granulomas due to infections and foreign antigens. Depending on the manifestations of different Type IV hypersensitivity diseases, there are different risk factors as well. Some diseases are more common in women such as autoimmune diseases, some are most common in men, such as allergic contact dermatitis.

DIAGNOSTICS

The diagnostic path includes various tests and clinical findings such as contact dermatitis test wherein inflammation occurs when the sensitizing chemical comes in contact with the skin surface. A variety of chemicals can cause this type of reaction. They include various drugs, excretions from certain plants, metals such as chromium, nickel and mercury, industrial products such as hair-dyes, cosmetics and resins. Another test is Tuberculin-test which is used to determine whether an individual has been infected with causative agent of tuberculosis (*Mycobacterium tuberculosis*) or not. In this test, small amount of protein extracted from Mycobacterium are injected into the skin. If the reactive T cells are present- redness and swelling will appear hence concluding that the test is positive. The diagnostic path may also include blood tests to assess the types and levels of blood cells present in the circulation as well as to detect the quantities of immunoglobulin. Allergy testing can also help in isolating the specific allergens.

TREATMENT

Type IV hypersensitivity diseases are usually long-standing and require on-going treatment if there is flaring up of diseases. However, it does not cause life-threatening conditions such as anaphylaxis or angioedema. Although Type IV hypersensitivity diseases can cause significant inconvenience in terms of their signs and symptoms, with good treatment plan the most of the diseases can be well controlled. Treatment options, either given alone or in combined form include the following:

- Allergen avoidance: prevention and avoidance of possible triggers are the mainstay of the treatment. However, this is impractical in some diseases such as allergic contact dermatitis because some of the substances cannot be identified and remained unknown for a long period of time. However, if known this is a useful and effective method for diseases with well-known allergen.
- Steroids: These drugs are used for late phase of reaction and they include Prednisolone, Dexamethasone, etc. Depending on the diseases, the steroid could become long term medication.
- Other immunosuppressive medications such as Methotrexate and Cyclosporine act through different mechanisms to achieve similar results.
- Various therapies are designed to reduce the inflammation caused by T cell mediated hypersensitivity reaction disorders using Corticosteroids, and antagonists against cytokines such as TNF and to inhibit T cell responses with immunosuppressive drugs. Many newer agents are being developed to inhibit T cell responses. These include; agents that block co-stimulators such as B7, and antagonists against receptors for cytokines such as IL2. There is also great hope for inducing tolerance in pathogenic cells, but no successful clinical trait has been reported yet.

Examples of Delayed Type Hypersensitivity Reaction

- *Contact sensitivity*

  It is often referred to as contact dermatitis and is a form of DTH in which the target organ is the skin, and the inflammatory response is produced as a result of contact with sensitizing substances on the skin surface. Thus, it is a primary epidermal reaction characterised by eczema at the site of contact with the allergen. Prototype for this form of DTH is poison ivy dermatitis.

- *Granulomatous hypersensitivity*

  Sometimes the antigen may be persistent, serving as a chronic source of stimulation. E.g., a parasite named *Schistosoma mansoni* produces schistostome eggs that induce granulomatous hypersensitivity. These may be present life-long in an individual. Under such circumstances, continuous accumulation of macrophages in circulation leads to clusters of epithelioid cells, which fuse to form giant cells in granulomas.
- *Tuberculin type hypersensitivity*

  These reactions are cutaneous inflammatory reactions characterised by an area of firm red swelling that is maximal at 48-72 hours after challenge.
- *Allograft rejection*

  It occurs when transplanted tissue (from an allogenic donor) is rejected by the recipient's immune system, which destroys the transplanted tissue.

It happens due to the genetic differences within the major histocompatibility complex (MHC) and hence results in T-cell mediated graft rejection.

CONCLUSION

Type IV hypersensitivity reaction is commonly referred to as Delayed type hypersensitivity (DTH) and it is the only hypersensitivity category that is purely cell-mediated, rather than antibody mediated. Delayed type hypersensitivity is an injurious cytokine-mediated inflammatory reaction resulting from the activation of T cells. The reaction is called hypersensitivity because It reflects excessive i.e., injurious immune responses and delayed because it typically develops during 24 to 48 hours after antigen challenge. Type IV reaction was described first by Robert Koch in 1890, he observed that the individuals infected with Mycobaterium tuberclosis, developed a localised inflammatory response when injected intradermally with a filtrate derived from a mycobacterial culture. He then called this localised skin reaction a, "tuberculin reaction". Contact dermatitis is an example of Type IV hypersensitivity reaction. DTH responses are responsible for granulomas associated with tuberculosis. DTH requires T cells to be sensitized to the antigen. Subsequent re-exposure to antigen results in cytokine generation, inflammation and recruitment of macrophages.

Multiple Choice Questions (MCQs)

1. Cell-mediated immune responses are

A. enhanced by depletion of complement.

B. suppressed by cortisone.

C. enhanced by depletion of T cells.

D. suppressed by antihistamine.

E. enhanced by depletion of macrophages.

2. The predominant antigen presenting cell in contact hypersensitivity (e.g., poison ivy) is the

A. T lymphocyte.

B. B lymphocyte.

C. basophil.

D. Langerhans cell.

E. NK cell.

3. The cutaneous response of delayed hypersensitivity

A. can be passively transferred by antibody.

B. shows erythema (redness) and induration 1–2 days after injection of the antigen.

C. depends upon the attachment of IgE antibody to mast cells.

D. is mediated by B lymphocytes.

4. Delayed hypersensitivity as typified by the Mantoux reaction to tuberculin is mediated by

A. lymphocytes.
B. polymorphonuclear cells.
C. anaphylactic antibodies.
D. complement binding antibodies.
E. antigen–antibody complexes.

5. The clinical disease most likely to involve a reaction to a hapten in its etiology is

A. systemic lupus erythematosus after treatment with glucocorticoids.
B. hemolytic anemia after treatment with penicillin.
C. juvenile diabetes after treatment with insulin.
D. rejection of kidney graft after treatment with cyclosporin.

6. Which hypersensitivity reactions are T cell mediated?

A. Type I
B. Type II
C. Type III
D. Type IV
E. None of these

7. Type IV hypersensitivity is mediated by?

A. T cells
B. Eosinophils
C. Erythrocytes
D. Neutrophils

8. Which of following does not involve cell-mediated immunity?

A. contact sensitivity to lipstick
B. rejection of a liver graft
C. serum sickness
D. tuberculin reaction

9. A positive delayed-type hypersensitivity skin reaction involves the interaction of:

A. Antigen, complement, and cytokines
B. Antigen, antigen-sensitive lymphocytes, and macrophages
C. Antigen —antibody complexes, complement, and neutrophils
D. IgE antibody, antigen, and mast cells

10. Delayed type hypersensitivity response occurs in:

A. 3 phases
B. 2 phases
C. Single phase
D. None of the above

11. Cytotoxic T cells (CTLs) generally recognize antigen in association with

A. class II MHC determinants
B. class I MHC determinants
C. class III MHC determinants
D. HLA-DR determinants

12. CD8 positive cells

A. can be classified into Th1 and Th2 subgroups based on their biological function.
B. do not produce IFNγ.
C. can recognize and kill virus infected cells.
D. can bind free virus.
E. do not require direct cell to cell contact with their targets for killing.

13. Th1 cells do not

A. express CD4.
B. produce IFNγ.
C. activate macrophages.
D. bind soluble antigen.

14. Which is most appropriate Statement about Macrophages:

A. circulate in the blood stream

B. produce nitric oxide

C. have receptors for IgM

D. are the first leukocytes to arrive at the site of a skin infection

E. are the main immune cells for dealing with viruses

15. Molecules involved in lymphocyte activation include all of the following EXCEPT

A. CD3

B. CD79b

C. CD14

D. lck

E. CD28

16. Graft survival can be enhanced *without* generalized immunosuppression by

A. matching for HLA antigen.

B. anti-thymocyte globulin.

C. cyclosporin A therapy.

D. steroids or cytotoxic drugs

ANSWER KEY:

1.B, 2.D, 3.B, 4.A, 5.B, 6.D, 7.A, 8.C, 9.B, 10.B, 11.B, 12.C, 13.D, 14.B, 15.C, 16.A

FREQUENTLY ASKED QUESTIONS (FAQS)

1. Define Delayed-type hypersensitivity reaction.

Answer: Type IV hypersensitivity reaction is commonly referred to as Delayed type hypersensitivity (DTH) and it is the only hypersensitivity category that is purely cell-mediated, rather than antibody mediated.

Delayed type hypersensitivity is an injurious cytokine-mediated inflammatory reaction resulting from the activation of T cells. The reaction is called hypersensitivity because It reflects excessive i.e., injurious immune responses and delayed because it typically develops during 24 to 48 hours after antigen challenge. Whereas antibody can be present in a preformed state, antigen-specific T cells need time to proliferate and then synthesize and secrete cytokines – hence referred to as "*Delayed Type Hypersensitivity*".

2. Outline the classification of Type IV hypersensitivity reaction?

Answer: Type IV reactions are subdivided into three categories based on the time of onset, the clinical manifestations, and the cells involved. The main features of the different categories in one such classification include:

- Tuberculin type reaction (seen as local induration): The antigen is presented intradermally and reaction time varies from 48–72 hours. The main cells involved are lymphocytes, monocytes, and macrophages.
- Contact type reaction (seen as eczema): This type of reaction occurs by cutaneous contact (e.g., with chemicals, poison ivy, nickel) and reaction time varies from 48–72 hours. The main cells involved are lymphocytes, macrophages.
- Granulomatous type reaction (as in leprosy): In this case antigen persists in the host and the reaction time varies from 21–28 days. The main cells involved are macrophages, epitheloid, and giant cells.

3. What treatment is adopted for Type IV hypersensitivity?

Answer: Certain cases of DTH reactions such as contact sensitivity and tuberculin reaction resolve after a period of days to weeks following removal of the antigen. Corticosteroids applied either topically or systematically constitute a very effective treatment for these forms of hypersensitivity. For other severe forms such as allograft rejection, immunosuppressive therapies are commonly used including treatment with drugs such as cyclosporine.

4. Give examples of each type of hypersensitivity reaction responses?

Answer: The example of Type I hypersensitivity reaction is – allergic rhinitis. The example of Type II hypersensitivity reaction is – transfusion reactions. The example of Type III hypersensitivity reaction is – serum sickness. The example of Type IV hypersensitivity reaction is – leprosy.

5. Who first described Type IV hypersensitivity reaction?

Answer: Type IV reaction was described first by Robert Koch in 1890, he observed that the individuals infected with Mycobaterium tuberclosis, developed a localised inflammatory response when injected intradermally with a filtrate derived from a mycobacterial culture. He then called this localised skin reaction a, "tuberculin reaction". In reference, to the delayed onset of the reaction and to the tissue damage (hypersensitivity) that is often associated with it, its name was changed to delayed-type or Type IV reaction.

6. Give examples of delayed-type hypersensitivity?

Answer: The following represent the examples of Delayed-type hypersensitivity. These are

- Contact sensitivity
- Granulomatous hypersensitivity
- Tuberculin type hypersensitivity
- Allograft rejection

7. Explain contact sensitivity.

Answer. It is often referred to as contact dermatitis and is a form of DTH in which the target organ is the skin, and the inflammatory response is produced as a result of contact with sensitizing substances on the skin surface. Thus, it is a primary epidermal reaction characterised by eczema at the site of contact with the allergen. Prototype for this form of DTH is poison ivy dermatitis.

8. Explain granulomatous hypersensitivity.

Answer: Sometimes the antigen may be persistent, serving as a chronic source of stimulation, e.g., a parasite named *Schistosoma mansoni* produces schistostome eggs that induce granulomatous hypersensitivity. These may be present life-long in an individual. Under such circumstances, continuous accumulation of macrophages in circulation leads to clusters of epithelioid cells, which fuse to form giant cells in granulomas.

9. Define Tuberculin type hypersensitivity

Answer: These reactions are cutaneous inflammatory reactions characterised by an area of firm red swelling that is maximal at 48-72 hours after challenge.

10. What is allograft rejection?

Answer: It occurs when transplanted tissue (from an allogenic donor) is rejected by the recipient's immune system, which destroys the transplanted tissue. It happens due to the genetic differences within the major histocompatibility complex (MHC) and hence results in T-cell mediated graft rejection.

11. How is Type IV hypersensitivity involved in pathogenesis?

Answer: Type IV hypersensitivity is involved in the pathogenesis of many autoimmune and infectious diseases such as tuberculosis, leprosy, blastomycosis, histoplasmosis, toxoplasmosis, Leishmaniasis etc. and granulomas due to infections and foreign antigens. Depending on the manifestations of different Type IV hypersensitivity diseases, there are different risk factors as well. Some diseases are more common in women such as autoimmune diseases, some are most common in men, such as allergic contact dermatitis.

12. Is Type IV hypersensitivity Antibody-mediated or cell-mediated response?

Answer: The Type IV hypersensitivity reaction is the only hypersensitivity that is cell-mediated hypersensitivity reaction.

13. Which cells are involved in mediating Type IV hypersensitivity reaction?

Answer. Once a Type IV response initiates, a number of non-specific cells and active mediators are set in to play, resulting in their enhanced amplification. Macrophages are the main effector cells of this response, with only the 5% involvement of antigen-specific T_H1 cells. Cytokine release induce blood monocytes to stick to endothelial cells and migrate into the surrounding tissue from blood. It is during this process, the monocytes differentiate into activated macrophages. These activated macrophages show increased levels of phagocytic activity and heightened release of lytic enzymes in the area of infection leading to non-specific destruction of cells and hence of the intracellular pathogen.

14. Treatment of Type IV hypersensitivity involves…

Answer: Treatment options, either given alone or in combined form include the following:

- *Allergen avoidance:* prevention and avoidance of possible triggers are the mainstay of the treatment. However, this is impractical in some diseases such as allergic contact dermatitis because some of the substances cannot be identified and remained unknown for a long period of time.
- *Steroids:* These drugs are used for late phase of reaction and they include Prednisolone, Dexamethasone, etc. Depending on the diseases, the steroid could become long term medication.
- *Other immunosuppressive medications* such as Methotrexate and Cyclosporine act through different mechanisms to achieve similar results.
- *Using Corticosteroids, and antagonists* against cytokines such as TNF and to inhibit T cell responses with immunosuppressive drugs. Many newer agents are being developed to inhibit T cell responses. These include; agents that block co-stimulators such as B7, and antagonists against receptors for cytokines such as IL2.

There is also great hope for inducing tolerance in pathogenic cells, but no successful clinical trait has been reported yet.

15. What Is Tuberculin-Test?

Answer: Tuberculin-test, is the test which is used to determine whether an individual has been infected with causative agent of tuberculosis (*Mycobacterium tuberculosis*) or not. In this test, small amount of protein extracted from Mycobacterium are injected into the skin. If the reactive T cells are present- redness and swelling will appear hence concluding that the test is positive.

ASSIGNMENTS:

Q1. Explain the concept of Type IV hypersensitivity.

Q2. Why is Type IV hypersensitivity called Delayed type hypersensitivity? Explain.

Q3. Describe contact sensitivity with examples.

Q4. Pen down few points of differences between contact sensitivity and tuberculin skin reaction.

Q5. Explain the process by which macrophages are activated.

REFERENCES

Askenase PW. Yes T cells, but three different T cells (αβ, γδ and NK T cells) and also B-1 cells mediate contact sensitivity. *Clin Exp Immunol* 2001;125:345–350.

Bean AGD, Roach DR, Briscoe H, et al. Structural deficiencies in granuloma formation in tumor necrosis factor gene-targeted mice underlie the heightened susceptibility to aerosol *Mycobacterium tuberculosis* infection which is not compensated for by lymphotoxin. *J Immunol* 1999;162:3504–3511.

Bjune G, Barnetson RStC, Ridley DS, et al. Lymphocyte transformation test in leprosy; correlation of the response with inflammation of lesions. *Clin Exp Immunol* 1976;25:85–94.

Britton WJ, Garsia RJ. Mycobacterial infections. In: Bradley J, McCluskey J, eds. *Clinical immunology,* vol. 38. London: Oxford University Press; 1997:483–498.

Britton WJ, Lockwood DN. *Leprosy. Lance*t 2004;363:1209–1219.

Casanova J-L, Abel L. Genetic dissection of immunity to mycobacteria: the human model. *Annu Rev Immunol* 2002;40:581–620.

Daniel H, Present MD, Rutgeerts P, et al. Infliximab for the treatment of fistulas in patients with Crohn's disease. *N Eng J Med* 1999;18:1398-1405.

Enk AH, Katz SI. Contact hypersensitivity as a model for T-cell activation in skin. *J Invest Dermatol* 1995;105:805-835.

Flynn JL, Chan J, Triebold KJ, et al. An essential role for interferon-γ in resistance to *Mycobacterium tuberculosis* infection. *J Exp Med* 1993;178:2249–2254.

Flynn JL, Chan J. Immunology of tuberculosis. *Annu Rev Immunol* 2001;19:93–129.

Girolomoni G, Sebastiani S, Albanesi C, Cavani A. T cell subpopulations in the development of atopic and contact allergy. *Curr Opin Immunol* 2001;13:733–737.

Grabbe S, Schwarz, T. Immunoregulatory mechanisms involved in elicitation of allergic contact hypersensitivity. *Immunol Today* 1998;19:37-43.

Kalish RS, Wood JA, LaPorte A. Processing of urushiol (poison ivy) hapten by both endogenous and exogenous pathways for presentation to T cells in vitro. *J Clin Invest* 1999;93:2039-2047.

Kindler V, Sappino A-P, Gran GE, et al. The inducing role of tumour necrosis factor in the development of bactericidal granulomas during BCG infection. *Cell* 1989;56:731-740.

Klimas N. Delayed hypersensitivity skin testing. In: *Manual of clinical laboratory immunology,* 5th edn. Washington: ASM Press;1997:276-280.

Roach DR, Bean AGD, Demangel C, et al. Tumor necrosis factor regulates chemokine induction essential for cell recruitment, granuloma formation and clearance of mycobacterial infection. *J Immunol* 2002;168:4620–4628.

Roach DR, Briscoe H, Saunders B, et al. *Secreted lymphotoxin-alpha is essential for the control of intracellular bacterial infection.*

Romagnani P, Annunziato F, Baccari M, et al. T cells and cytokines in Crohn's disease. *Curr Opin Immunol* 1997;9:793–799.

Salgame P. Host innate and TH1 responses and the bacterial factors that contain *Mycobacterium tuberculosis* infection. *Curr Opin Immunol* 2005;17:374-380.

Trinchieri G. Interleukin-12: a cytokine at the interface of inflammation and immunity. *Adv Immunol 1*998;70:133–195.

Von Andrian UH, Mackay CR. T cell function and migration: two sides of the same coin. *N Engl J Med* 2000;343:1020–1034.

Wallis RS, Broder MS, Wong JY, et al. Granulomatous infectious disease associated with tumor necrosis factor. *Clin Infect Dis* 2004;38:1261–1265.

Wang B, Eshe C, Mamelak A, et al. Cytokine knockouts in contact hypersensitivity research. *Cytokine Growth Factor Rev* 2003;14:381–389.

In: The Fundamentals of Hypersensitivities … ISBN: 978-1-53617-012-2
Editor: Manzoor Ahmad Mir © 2020 Nova Science Publishers, Inc.

Chapter 7

AEROALERGENS AND THEIR CONTROL

Nissar A. Wani, Bashir A. Sheikh, Safura Nisar, Umar Mehraj, Syed Suhail, Hina Qayoom and Manzoor Ahmad Mir*

Department of Bioresources, School of Biological Sciences, University of Kashmir, Srinagar J&K, India

ABSTRACT

Aeroallergens are airborne substances that can cause allergic reactions in sensitive individuals. They may be any substance light enough to be carried away by the air currents and capable of evoking an immune response. Aeroallergens can be of plant, animal or microbial origin. The most common indoor allergens are derived from dust mites, wild rodents, pets like cats and dogs, etc. Some aeroallergens are found only in a particular region while others seem to be ubiquitous. The frequency, variation and aerial transport depend on many factors. Many people who have inhaled allergies only experience symptoms during certain seasons. Pollen, grass, mold are most triggers of seasonal allergies. Changes in climate factors can effect aeroallergen production, which in turn effects the severity of allergic illness through sensitivity

* Corresponding Author's Email: drmanzoor@kashmiruniversity.ac.in.

and response pathways. Aeroallergens include a variety of plant and animal material, usually protein. The common types of aeroallergens are-pollen, dust mites, pet dander, mold spores. The most common allergic conditions include-allergic rhinitis (hay fever), asthma, allergic conjunctivitis, allergic bronchitis, allergic eczema.

Keywords: aeroallergens, asthma, allergic conjunctivitis, hay fever, eczema, antihistamines

OBJECTIVES

- Define Aeroallergens?
- Discuss the effect of climate change on aeroallergens production
- Describe different types of aeroallergens.
- Discuss the effects of aeroallergens & the allergies caused by them
- Various diagnostic tests employed for detecting aero-allergy.
- Discuss the prevention and control of aeroallergens.

INTRODUCTION

Aeroallergens are airborne substances that can cause allergic reactions in sensitive individuals. They may be any substance light enough to be carried away by the air currents and capable of evoking an immune response. Aeroallergens can be of plant, animal or microbial origin. Plant source aeroallergens are mainly outdoors while as animal source are most relevant indoors. Aeroallergens like pollens, spores, etc. stimulate immune reaction in a sensitive person. Airborne particles like tree and grass pollens induce allergic response like allergic rhinitis in sensitized people. Clinically significant aeroallergens are proteins or glycoproteins with a molecular weight of 10KD to 60KD. Indoor allergens are present inside buildings and given the chronic nature of the exposures, indoor allergies tend to the development of asthma. The most common indoor allergens are derived from dust mites, wild rodents, pets like cats and dogs, etc. Some aeroallergens are found only in a particular region while others seem to be ubiquitous. The frequency, variation and aerial transport depend on many factors. Regional surveys of aeroallergens and their aerobiology are necessary in order to efficiently treat the sufferers and prepare relevant extracts. The children are mostly affected by aeroallergens than adults. The most common aeroallergens are the pollens of wind pollinated plants and ragweed pollen is most common among the group. Ragweed pollen is the cause of more than 90 percent of pollonosis in the United States (Figure 7.1).

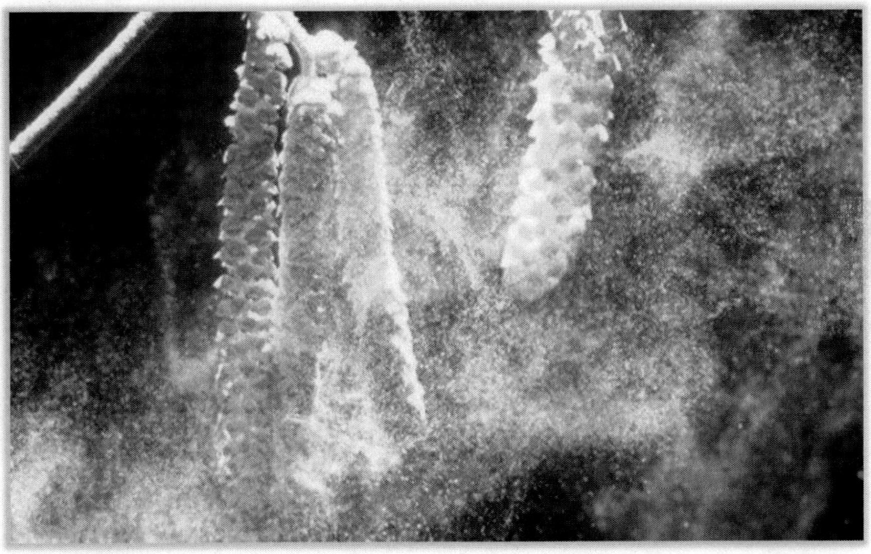

Figure 7.1. Pollens from different plants, act as aeroallergens.

Every individual is not allergic to the allergen, but the individuals that become sensitized by initial exposures to the allergen show acute allergic symptoms on subsequent exposures (Figure 7.2). The effects of aeroallergens on human health are not adverse in most of the individuals but in some individual's severe symptoms of bronchial asthma may occur.

Allergic reactions caused by aeroallergens are known as inhaled allergies. These are the most common type of allergy. Symptoms may include

- Sneezing
- Runny nose
- Itchy eyes
- Watery eyes.

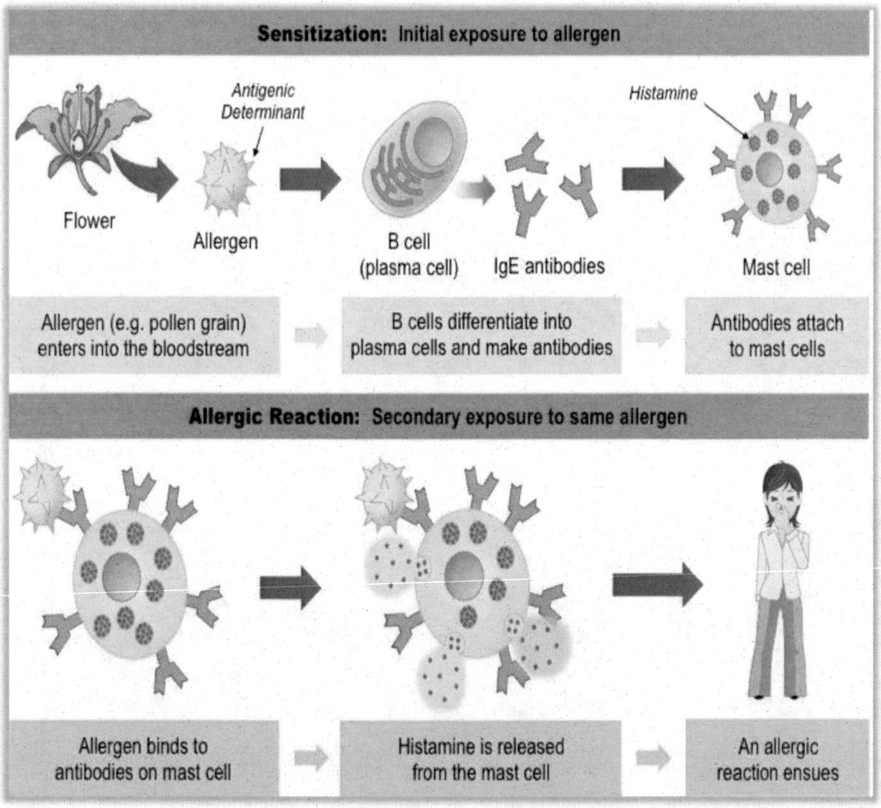

Figure 7.2. Representing the prior exposure of an individual to an allergen, causing an allergic reaction on second exposure.

Many people who have inhaled allergies only experience symptoms during certain seasons. Pollen, grass, mold are most triggers of seasonal allergies. Pollen is a fine powder that comes from trees, weeds and grass.

Each season beginning in the spring and continuing through fall, the amount of pollen in the air increases. This increase may trigger symptoms in people sensitive to pollen. Avoiding pollen isn't always as simple as retreating inside during allergy season.

Other types of airborne allergens are prevalent indoors. These include: Fungi, Mold, Pet dander and Dust mites.

EFFECT OF CLIMATE CHANGE ON AEROALLERGEN PRODUCTION

Changes in climate factors can effect aeroallergen production, which in turn effects the severity of allergic illness through sensitivity and response pathways. For example, greater pollen concentrations in the air increase the chance of sensitization and subsequent aggravation of illness.

Exposure to higher concentrations of aeroallergens may lead to more severe allergic responses. Increased precipitations and temperature also play an important role in increased production of pollens. Increased carbon dioxide concentration in the atmosphere acts as a fertilizer for plant growth. The fertilizing effects of carbon dioxide, as well as increased temperatures from climate change, increase pollen production and the allergen content of pollen grains. In addition, higher temperatures change the timing and duration of the pollen season. As the local climate of area change, plants move their pollen and spore into new areas therefore introducing people to allergens to which they have not been exposed previously. Severe weather conditions such as thunderstorms provide fascinating evidence of connection between weather, aeroallergens and allergic diseases. Higher rates of asthma attacks have been reported during thunderstorms, not only in the individuals which were asthmatic but for the individuals who previously had only allergic rhinitis. Thunderstorm winds provide the favorable conditions for pollen grains to burst and release allergen particles small enough to enter the lower airways. By mitigating effects of climate change like decreasing greenhouse gas emission and reduce other air pollutants result in the decrease in respiratory diseases and allergies. Aeroallergens cause seasonal as well as perennial allergies. Seasonal allergies are caused by the allergens which are present at that particular season like pollen grains. Perennial allergies are caused by the allergens that are present throughout the year like dust mites, occupational aeroallergens, etc.

Different Types of Aeroallergens

Airborne allergens present in the atmosphere induce allergic reactions in an individual who are sensitized. They are also called as inhalant allergens they are harmless to people which are not allergic. Aeroallergens include a variety of plant and animal material, usually protein. The common types of aeroallergens are:

- Pollen.
- Dust mites.
- Pet dander.
- Mold spores.

Pollen

Plants produce very small particles which are not visible to the naked eye for the purpose of reproduction. These tiny particles are known as pollens. In some species, the plants use the pollen from its own flowers to fertilize itself whereas in some species pollens from other flowers are used for pollination. These pollens need to be transferred from one flower to another, this is done by the help of insects and wind which act as carriers for these pollens. These pollens are small, lightweight and dry and can be easily carried away by wind (Figure 7.3). These pollens remain present in the air behave as allergen and causes allergies when inhaled. Pollen allergens are one of the main causes of type I allergies affecting up to 30% of the population. Aero allergenic pollen grains are mainly contributed from the plants belonging to the family Poaceae, Chenopodiaceae, Amaranthaceae and Asteraceae. Occurrence and abundance of pollen grains in the environment differ according to season and vegetation types. Pollen most commonly triggers seasonal allergies. Grasses are the most common cause of allergy. Weed pollen including sagebrush, pigweed, lamb's quarters and tumbleweed also trigger allergic reactions. Pollens usually cause seasonal allergic rhinitis. The amount of pollens present in the air is known as pollen count.

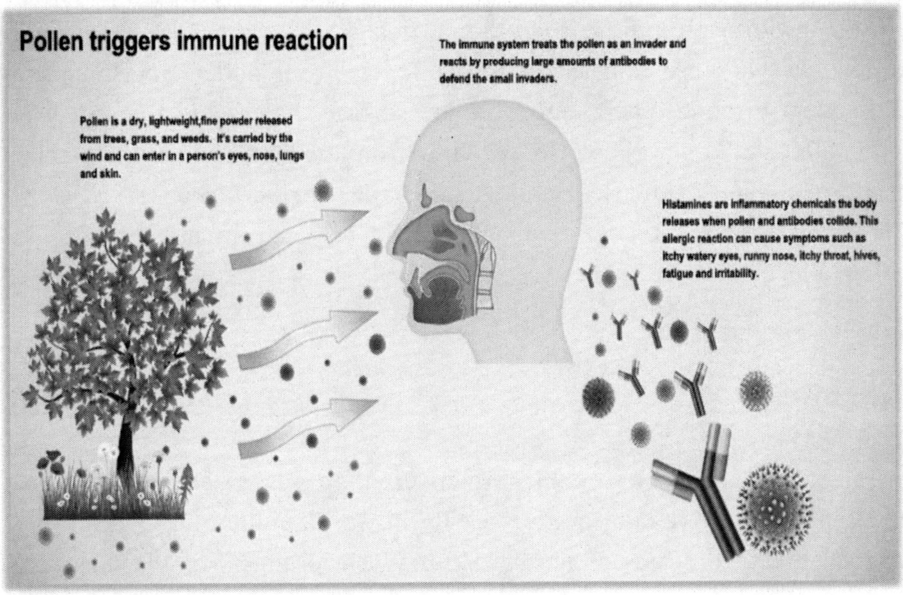

Figure 7.3. Representing pollens from different plant families, initiating allergic responses and playing main role in evoking type I allergic reaction.

People with pollen allergies only have symptoms when the pollens they are allergic to are present in the air. The symptoms include:

- Runny nose and mucous production.
- Itchy nose, eyes, ears and mouth.

- Sneezing.
- Stuffy nose (nasal congestion).
- Red and watery eyes.
- Swelling around the eyes.

Certain trees belonging to order Fagales, Lamiales, Proteales and Pinales produce pollens which are highly allergic. Pollen allergens are considered a major risk factor for both seasonal allergic rhinitis and asthma. Allergenic proteins are usually located within the pollen protoplast and readily released during rehydration process in some tree pollens. In trees like birch the allergens are located within the pollen cytoplasm, mostly in close proximity to ribosome-rich areas. Upon hydration, birch pollen allergens are released within minutes from pollen apertures and subsequently found on the entire pollen surface. Allergenic trees may be found almost all over the world, reaching from the temperate climate zones of Europe, North America, and Asia to the Mediterranean area, North Africa, the Indian subcontinent, whereas in tropical climate regions tree pollen allergies are virtually absent.

Dust Mites

Dust mites are microscopic organisms that are present in the house dust. Dust mites live and multiply easily in warm and humid places. They feed on the shed scales of human skin. Waste products of the dust mite produce allergic reactions. Dust mites thrive in temperatures of 68 to 77 degrees Fahrenheit. They also like humidity levels of 70 to 80 percent. They are well adapted to the environment inside our homes. They feed mainly on the tiny flakes of human skin that people shed each day. These flakes work their ways deep into the inner layers of furniture, carpets, bedding, stuffed toys, etc. The mites thrive at these places. An adult person shed up to 1.5 grams of skin in a day which is enough to feed one million dust mites. Dust mites are divided into two groups, house dust mites (HDMs) and storage mites (SMs), these two groups have been found in the household environment. Both the groups can induce airway inflammation through activation of innate and adaptive immunity and lead to asthma. There are many species of dust mites present in and around the houses. The two most common house dust mites are *Dermatophagoide pteronyssinus (Dp) and Dermatophgoides farina*. Two common storage mites (SMs) are *Blomia tropicalis (Bt), Turophapus puterscentias (Tp).* Dust mites are a common cause of asthma in children. A house which is visibly clean may trigger a dust mite allergic reaction because the particles are too tiny to be visible to naked eye and often cannot be removed by using normal cleaning procedures. A vigorous cleaning can make an allergic person's symptoms worse. Common dust mite allergy symptoms include:

- Sneezing.
- Runny nose.
- Itchy nose, mouth and throat.
- Stuffy nose.
- Itchy skin.
- Postnasal drip (a flow of mucus from behind nose into the throat).
- Cough.

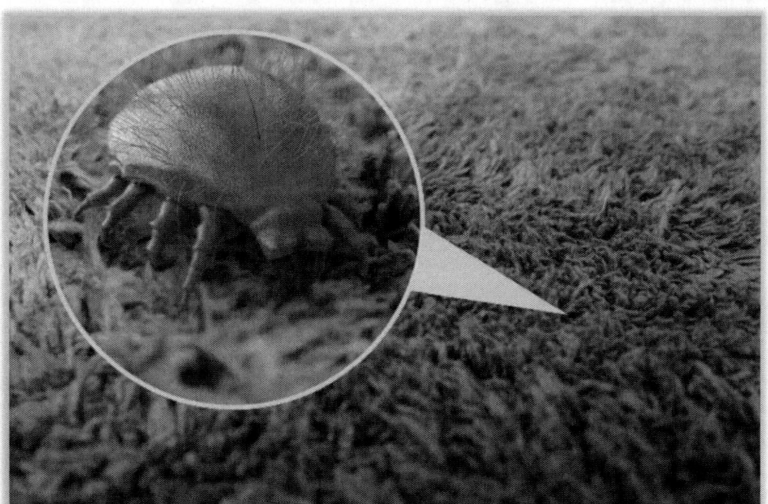

Figure 7.4. Showing the highlighted view of microscopic dust mite present in indoors, which is respsonsible for evoking allergic response.

Pet Dander

Pet dander is composed of tiny, even microscopic, flecks of skin shed cats, dogs, rodents, birds and other animals with fur or feathers. These bits of skin can cause reactions in people who are specifically allergic to these triggers. Animals secrete a number of proteins in their urine, sweat and saliva. The dried saliva, sweat, urine containing allergens may flake off in the air and become airborne. When it is inhaled by the allergic person, it triggers allergic reactions there.

Cat dander is the most common inhaled allergen source after house dust mite and pollen. Other animals and birds commonly kept as pets, such as parrot, rabbit, dogs also cause allergic reactions. Pet allergens are widely distributed in air because of their light weight and remain suspended in air for several hours before settling.

Pet dander is very sticky and remain attached to the body, hairs, clothes of the owner of the pet for long period of time and travels to them to other places. Male cats shed more allergen than females and cat shed more allergen than dogs.

Parrots also produce dander which can seriously affect the indoor air quality. The dander produced by the parrot is known as feather dust. This dander is produced from the feathers when they flap their wings or when they preen. Most of the birds have their preening gland located at the back of the base of the tail. When a bird preen itself, secretions from this gland spread all over the feathers. This dander is sticky and hard to remove. Some species of parrot also produce an additional type of feather dander that is called powder. This type of dander comes from the specialized feathers, which shed a fine waxy, white powder composed of protein keratin. Parrot dander of both the types trigger allergic reactions. Pet dander allergy include following symptoms:

- Facial pain
- Skin rash
- Coughing, shortness of breath and tightness of chest

- Sneezing
- Watery, red, itchy eyes

Mold Spores

Molds are fungi that can be found both indoors and outdoors. Molds grow best in warm, damp, and humid conditions, and spread and reproduce by making spores. Mold spores can survive harsh environmental conditions, such as dry conditions, that do not support normal mold growth. Some people are sensitive to molds; exposure of these people to molds can lead to symptoms such as stuffy nose and red or itchy eyes, or skin. Some people, such as those with allergies to molds or with asthma, may have more intense reactions. Severe reactions may occur among workers exposed to large amounts of molds in occupational settings, such as farmers working around moldy hay. Severe reactions may include fever and shortness of breath.

Molds are found in virtually every environment and can be detected, both indoors and outdoors, year round. Mold growth is encouraged by warm and humid conditions. Outdoors they can be found in shady, damp areas or places where leaves or other vegetation is decomposing. Indoors they can be found where humidity levels are high, such as basements or showers. The common types of molds found indoors are; Cladosporium, Penicillium, Alternaria, Aspergillus.

There are other substances which may sometimes induce allergy like reactions but does not qualify for aeroallergens. For example, smoke. Smoke has not been proven an allergen, but it is certainly an irritant, especially to people who are suffering from asthma or from allergic rhinitis. Cigarette smoke, both from smoking and from passive smoking, is known to increase the risk of allergic rhinitis and asthma. Children are especially vulnerable. Tobacco smoke releases thousands of toxic chemicals and irritants into the air, and anyone in the path of these tiny particles can be exposed. To be a true allergen, however, a particle must trigger cells in the immune system to release a cascade of inflammatory chemicals. Tobacco smoke is more accurately an irritant that can produce allergy-like reactions. Children and adults who are already compromised with allergies or allergic asthma may be particularly sensitive to smoke around them. Tobacco smoke gets into the allergic person's airways and weakens the protective lining of cells there, making it easier for true allergens to penetrate the lungs.

Effects of Aeroallergens and Allergies Caused by Them

When an aeroallergen enters the body an inappropriate immune response is generated against it. The inappropriate immune response is known as allergy. The allergies can occur at any age; the risk of developing allergies is genetic. It is related toone's family history of allergy. If neither of the parents is allergic, the chance for allergies is about 15%. If one parent is allergic, the risk increases to 30% and if both are allergic, the risk is greater than 60%.

Allergens cause the production of immunoglobulin E, an antibody that is present in every individual in small amounts. Allergic persons, however, produce immunoglobulin E in abnormally quantities. Normally, this antibody is important in protecting an individual from parasites, but not from other allergens. During the sensitization period in allergy, immunoglobulin E is overproduced. It coats certain potentially explosive cells that contain chemicals including histamine. These chemicals, in turn, cause inflammation and the typical allergic symptoms. This is how the immune system becomes misguided and primed to cause an allergic reaction when stimulated by an allergen.

The most common allergic conditions include

- Allergic rhinitis (hay fever).
- Asthma.
- Allergic conjunctivitis.
- Allergic bronchitis.
- Allergic eczema.

Allergic Rhinitis

Allergic rhinitis is inflammation of inside of the nose caused by an allergen, such as pollen, dust, mold, or flakes of skin from certain animals. It is an IgE-mediated allergic reaction that affects the upper respiratory tract. It is also known as hay fever. It gives rise to symptoms such as nasal congestion, sinus headache, runny nose, watery eyes, itching and sneezing. There are two types of hay fever: seasonal and chronic hay fever.

Seasonal hay fever is caused by pollen: tree pollen in spring, grass pollen in summer, and weed pollen in autumn. Chronic rhinitis is a year-round problem, and is often caused by dust and animal dander in addition to pollens that may exist at the time.

Common symptoms of allergic rhinitis include

- sneezing
- runny nose
- coughing
- dark circles under eyes
- frequent headaches
- excessive fatigue.

Children can develop allergic rhinitis too, and it typically appears before the age of 10. The symptoms in children are similar to those in adults. Children usually develop watery, bloodshot eyes, shortness of breath.

Treatment of Allergic Rhinitis

Allergic rhinitis can be treated in several ways. These include medications, as well as home remedies and possibly alternative medicines.

Antihistamines can be used to treat allergies. They work by stopping body from making histamine. Some popular anti histamines are

- fexofenadine
- diphenhydramine
- levocetirizine.

Decongestants can be used over a short time usually no longer than three days, to relieve a stuffy nose and sinus pressure. Using them for a longer time can cause a rebound effect, meaning once use of decongestants is stopped the symptoms will actually get worse. Some of the common decongestants that can be used are

- Oxymetazoline
- pseudoephedrine
- phenylpherine.

Asthma

Asthma is a severe form of respiratory allergy that produces contraction of the trachea and bronchi. Asthma attacks can be brought about on by aeroallergens. Asthma is a syndrome with three cardinal features- generalized but reversible airways obstruction, bronchial hyper-responsiveness, airways inflammation. In allergic asthma reactions, constriction of the smooth muscles brings about a progressive closure of the airways. The inability to fill the lungs with air can cause serious complications. Asthma results from complex interactions between an individual's inherited genetic makeup and their interactions with the environment. The factors that cause a genetically predisposed individual to become asthmatic is not fully understood.

The following are risk factors for asthma:

- Family history of allergic conditions
- Personal history of hay fever
- Viral respiratory illness during childhood
- Exposure to cigarette smoke.

When the breathing passages become irritated or infected, an attack is triggered. The attack may come on suddenly or develop slowly over several days or hours. The main symptoms that signal an attack are as follows

- wheezing,
- breathlessness
- chest tightness
- coughing
- difficulty speaking

Symptoms may occur during the day or at night. If they happen at night, they may disturb sleep. Wheezing is the most common symptom of an asthma attack. Wheezes are most often heard during exhalation, but they can occur during breathing in (inhaling).

Not all asthmatics wheeze, and not all people who wheeze are asthmatics.

Treatment of Asthma

Antihistamines are not effective in the treatment of asthmatic attacks, hence drugs like epinephrine, corticosteroids and cromolyn sodium have proved beneficial in treating allergic asthma attacks.

Allergic Conjunctivitis

Allergic conjunctivitis is an eye inflammation caused by an allergic reaction to substances like pollen, dust or mold spores. The eye becomes sore and inflamed. Symptoms occur because the overreacting immune system makes the body release histamine and other active substances through mast cells. The blood vessels dilate, or expand, and this irritates the nerve endings. The result is an increased secretion of tears. The inside of the eyelid and eyeball have a membrane called the conjunctiva. The conjunctiva is susceptible to irritation from allergens. The following allergens that cause conjunctivitis are pollen, dust, animal fur, make up.

Allergic conjunctivitis is of two types:

- Acute allergic conjunctivitis

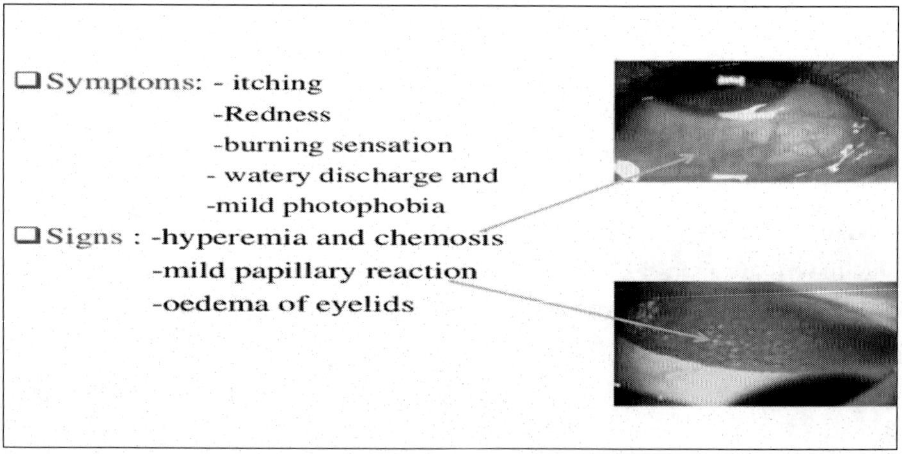

Figure 7.5. Showing the symptoms of conjunctivitis affected eye.

This is more common in allergy seasons and is a short-term condition. In this condition eyelids swell, itch and burn.

- Chronic allergic conjunctivitis

It is the less common condition and occur throughout the year. It is the milder response to allergens like dust and animal dander. Common symptoms include burning and itching of eyes and light sensitivity.

Symptoms of allergic conjunctivitis include (Figure 7.5):

- Red or pink eyes: The eyes become irritated as the capillaries, or small blood vessels, widen in the conjunctiva.
- Swollen eyelids: The eyelids may puff up when the conjunctiva becomes inflamed, or if the person may have been rubbing them a lot.
- Pain: This affect one or both eyes.
- Itchiness: As the eyes are irritated, they may itch. Rubbing can make the itchiness worse.

Allergic Bronchitis

Bronchitis is inflammation or swelling of bronchial tubes that carry air to the lungs. Allergic bronchitis is caused by exposure to tobacco smoke, pollution, or dust. Allergic bronchitis is often called chronic bronchitis and is considered a type of chronic obstructive pulmonary disease (COPD). In bronchitis airways also produce too much mucus. Mucus normally protect lungs by trapping dust, bacteria and other particles before they get in. Large amount of mucus makes it harder to breath. Symptoms of allergic bronchitis include- productive cough, wheezing, chest tightness, tiredness. Bronchitis can also lead to certain complications. For example, lung infections such as pneumonia are possible. In the most severe cases, pneumonia can lead to an infection in the bloodstream called septicemia, which is often life-threatening.

Treatment for allergic bronchitis may include the following bronchodilators, steroids and oxygen therapy are some of the treatment options available for allergic bronchitis. People with severe allergic bronchitis may have decreased blood oxygen levels. If oxygen levels are low, oxygen therapy is recommended.

Allergic Eczema

Eczema is a reaction pattern that the skin produces in a number of diseases. It is a particular type of inflammatory reaction of the skin in which there is erythema (reddening), edema (swelling), papules (bumps) and crusting of the skin followed, finally, by thickening and scaling of the skin.

Eczema characteristically causes itching and burning of the skin. There are many distinct types of skin conditions that produce eczema including.

- Atopic dermatitis (chronic skin disease) is characterized by itchy, inflamed skin.
- Irritant contact eczema localized reaction that includes redness, itching and burning where the skin has come into contact with an irritant such as an acid, a cleaning agent, or other chemical.
- Stasis dermatitis after repeated exposure to the same allergen the body's immune recognition system becomes activated at the site of the next exposure and produced a dermatitis.
- Nummular eczema coin shaped areas of irritated skin most commonly on the arms, back, buttocks, and lower legs that may be crusted, scaling, and extremely itchy
- Neurodermatitis scaly patches of skin on the head, lower legs, wrists, or forearms caused by a localized itch (such as an insect bite) that becomes intensely irritated when scratched.
- Seborrheic eczema is a form of skin inflammation unknown cause that presents as yellowish, oily, scaly areas of skin on the scalp, face and occasionally other parts of the body.

DIAGNOSTIC TESTS FOR ALLERGIC REACTIONS

Diagnosis of Asthma

A person may be given lung (pulmonary) function tests to determine how much air moves in and out as the person breathe. These tests may include:

- *Spirometry*. This test estimates the narrowing of bronchial tubes by checking how much air a person can exhale after a deep breath and how fast it can breathe out.
- *Peak flow*. A peak flow meter is a simple device that measures how hard a person can breathe out. Lower than usual peak flow readings are a sign that lungs may not be working as well and that asthma may be getting worse.

Lung function tests often are done before and after taking a medication called a bronchodilator, such as albuterol, to open the airways. If lung function improves with use of a bronchodilator, it's likely that a person is having asthma.

Other tests to diagnose asthma include:

- *Methacholine challenge*. Methacholine is a known asthma trigger that, when inhaled, will cause mild constriction of airways. If the person reacts to the methacholine, the person is likely to have asthma. This test may be used even if the person's initial lung function test is normal.
- *Allergy testing*. This can be performed by a skin test or blood test. Allergy tests can identify allergy to pets, dust, mold and pollen. If important allergy triggers are identified, this can lead to a recommendation for allergen immunotherapy.
- *Sputum eosinophils*. This test looks for certain white blood cells (eosinophils) in the mixture of saliva and mucus (sputum) the person discharges during coughing. Eosinophils are present when symptoms develop and become visible when stained with a rose-colored dye (eosin).

Diagnosis of Allergic Rhinitis

Allergic rhinitis is usually confirmed when medical treatment starts. If a person responds well to antihistamines, it's almost certain that the person's symptoms are caused by an allergy. If the exact cause of allergic rhinitis is uncertain, individuals GP may refer him/her to a hospital allergy clinic for allergy testing.

The two main allergy diagnostic tests for allergic rhinitis are:

- *skin prick test* – where the allergen is placed on an individual's arm and the surface of the skin is pricked with a needle to introduce the allergen to individual's immune system; if the individual is allergic to the substance, a small itchy spot (welt) will appear
- *blood test* – to check for the immunoglobulin E (IgE) antibody in the individual's blood; individual's immune system produces this antibody in response to a suspected allergen.

Diagnosis of Allergic Bronchitis

Some of the common tests employed for diagnosis of Allergic bronchitis are:

- *Chest X-ray*. A chest X-ray can help determine if an individual has pneumonia or another condition that may explain the individual's cough. This is especially important if the individual ever was or currently is a smoker.
- *Sputum tests*. Sputum is the mucus that an individual cough up from his/her lungs. It can be tested to see if an individual has illnesses that could be helped by antibiotics. Sputum can also be tested for signs of allergies.

- *Pulmonary function test.* During a pulmonary function test, a person blows into a device called a spirometer, which measures how much air the person's lungs can hold and how quickly the person can get air out of his/her lungs. This test checks for signs of asthma or emphysema.

Diagnosis of Allergic Eczema

Eczema allergic condition is usually done by Patch test and Biopsy which are discussed here.

Patch Test

During this test, patches that contain common allergens are placed on the back of an individual. These patches remain in place for 48 hours. The patches are then removed and symptoms of an allergic reaction are checked. The skin is checked again after two more days to see if the individual has a delayed allergic reaction.

Biopsy

Other tests will be needed if it is difficult to make a diagnosis based on the patch test. Skin lesion biopsy is performed to make sure another health condition isn't causing the skin condition. During the biopsy a small sample of the affected skin is removed and is then sent to a laboratory for testing.

Prevention and Control of Aeroallergens

Controlling Indoor Allergens

There are two general approaches to the control of indoor allergens. One can attempt to control the sources (e.g., the dust mites, cats, cockroaches, etc.), or one can attempt to remove the allergens (e.g., the actual proteins that cause sensitization). Some of the measures to control the indoor allergens are:

- Remove all carpeting and minimize its use especially in kitchens and bedrooms.
- Minimize the use of upholstered furniture.
- Vacuum regularly with the sensitive person not doing the vacuuming.
- Chemical treatments have also been used for the reduction of dust mite allergens in carpeting.
- Washing of bedding in hot water continues to be recommended for control of dust mite allergen, although controlled trials have not been done to evaluate efficacy at preventing symptoms.

Almost any animal, fungus or plant can release allergens into the indoor environment. In order to decide on a remediation protocol, the nature of the source and the dynamics of allergen dispersal need to be considered. For mammals, allergen is generally contained in skin secretions, saliva, and/or urine. For arthropods, feces and eggs may contain the allergen, or secretions may be at fault. For many plants, the majority of allergens are contained in pollen. In each of these cases, exposure prevention involves removing the source, or somehow blocking the pathway of the allergen. In domestic environments, removal of sources is by far the best approach to reducing allergen exposure.

Controlling Outdoor Allergens

Use Portable Room Air Filters to Remove Allergens and Irritants from the Air

Look for devices that have HEPA filters. Clean or replace the filters according to the manufacturer's recommendations so as to get the very best results and keep air as clean as possible.

Dehumidify Your Space to Prevent Mold Growth

Mold is an infamous problem-causing allergen in the home. Though it looks stationary, mold can float easily through the air. Using a dehumidifier helps eliminate the moisture that feeds its growth in bathrooms, basements and other moisture-prone places in the home.

Keep Your Pets Clean

Dander and down from cats, dogs and birds feed dust mites in the home. And even though they don't mean to, animals bring outdoor allergens inside after a long day of play. To cut back on pet-related airborne allergens, wash pet bedding weekly and wipe down pets when they come inside.

Abstain from Outside Activities

If possible, during times of high pollen counts (if you are sensitive to pollens). The peak pollination occurs at different times of the day for different plants (for example, ragweed in the late morning, grasses in the afternoon).

CONCLUSION

Aeroallergens are airborne substances that can cause allergic reactions in sensitive individuals. They may be any substance light enough to be carried away by the air currents and capable of evoking an immune response. Aeroallergens can be of plant, animal or microbial origin. Plant source aeroallergens are mainly outdoors while as animal source are most relevant indoors. Aeroallergens like pollens, spores, etc. stimulate immune reaction in a sensitive person. Airborne particles like tree and grass pollens induce allergic response like allergic rhinitis in sensitized people. When an aeroallergen enters the body an inappropriate immune response is generated against it. The inappropriate immune response is known as allergy. The allergies can occur at any age; the risk of developing allergies is genetic. Pollen is a fine powder that comes from trees, weeds and grass.

Each season beginning in the spring and continuing through fall, the amount of pollen in the air increases. This increase may trigger symptoms in people sensitive to pollen. Molds are found in virtually every environment and can be detected, both indoors and outdoors, year round.

Mold growth is encouraged by warm and humid conditions. Outdoors they can be found in shady, damp areas or places where leaves or other vegetation is decomposing. There are other substances which may sometimes induce allergy like reactions but does not qualify for aeroallergens. For example, smoke. Smoke has not been proven an allergen, but it is certainly an irritant, especially to people who are suffering from asthma or from allergic rhinitis. Cigarette smoke, both from smoking and from passive smoking, is known to increase the risk of allergic rhinitis and asthma. There are two general approaches to the control of indoor allergens. One can attempt to control the sources (e.g., the dust mites, cats, cockroaches, etc.), or one can attempt to remove the allergens (e.g., the actual proteins that cause sensitization).

MULTIPLE CHOICE QUESTIONS (MCQS)

1. A positive blood test for allergy must include:

A. Antibodies
B. Gluten
C. Antioxidants
D. Enzymes

2. An allergic reaction can produce urticaria. A common term for urticaria is

A. Atopic dermatitis
B. Eczema
C. Folliculitis
D. Hives

3. Allergies can best be described as

A. Sneezing, itching, watery eyes, scratchy throat

B. An overreaction from the immune system to a foreign substance

C. The onset of a cold during spring months

D. A reaction to the influenza virus during spring months

4. Which of these occupations is at risk for developing latex allergy

A. Health care workers

B. Glove manufacturing workers, laboratory technicians

C. Estheticians, greenhouse workers

D. All of the above

5. The diagnosis of allergic contact dermatitis can be confirmed by

A. Tzanck preparation

B. KOH examination

C. Patch testing

D. Wood's lamp examination

6. To determine if a patient is allergic to rye grass, the best test to perform is

A. Total IgE testing

B. Skin prick test

C. DAT

D. Complement fixation

7. Atopic dermatitis is also called often called

A. Acne

B. Eczema

C. Psoriasis

D. Hives

8. Rheumatoid arthritis is an ____ disease that affects the ____

A. Allergic/cartilage

B. Autoimmune/nerves

C. Autoimmune/joints

D. Immunodeficiency/muscles
E. Allergic/muscles

9. Which of the following is considered an autoimmune disease?
A. Rheumatoid arthritis
B. AIDS
C. SCID
D. Agammaglobulinemia

10. The typical sequence of events in an allergic reaction is as follows
A. The allergen combines with the circulating IgE, then the IgE-allergen complex binds to the mast cells
B. The allergen binds to the IgE fixed to mast cells
C. The allergen is processed by antigen-presenting cells and then binds to histamine receptors
D. The allergen is binds to IgG

11. Which of the following is the gold standard for asthma management?
A. Antihistamines
B. Corticosteroids
C. Adhesion molecule antagonists
D. Epinephrine

12. **Pollen would most likely evoke which of the following type of** hypersensitivity reaction?
A. Type I hypersensitivity
B. Cytotoxic hypersensitivity
C. Delayed type hypersensitivity
D. Type III hypersensitivity

13. Atopic dermatitis is an example of

A. Type IV hypersensitivity
B. Cytotoxic hypersensitivity
C. Immediate type hypersensitivity
D. Type III hypersensitivity

14. **Which among the following is not an aeroallergen**.
A. Dust mite
B. Pollen
C. Cockroach calyx
D. Mold spore

15. **Symptoms of allergic conjunctivitis include**
A. Red or pink eyes
B. Swelling in eyes
C. All of the above
D. None of the above

ANSWER KEY:

1.A, 2.D, 3.B, 4.D, 5.C, 6.B, 7.B, 8.C, 9.A, 10.B, 11.B, 12.A, 13.C, 14.C, 15.C

FREQUENTLY ASKED QUESTIONS (FAQS)

1. **What are aeroallergens?**

Answer: Aeroallergens are airborne substances that can cause allergic reactions in sensitive individuals. They may be any substance light enough to be carried away by the air currents and capable of evoking an immune response. Aeroallergens can be of plant, animal or microbial origin. Plant source aeroallergens are mainly outdoors while as animal source are most relevant indoors. Aeroallergens like pollens, spores, etc. stimulate immune reaction in a sensitive person. Airborne particles like tree and grass pollens induce allergic response like allergic rhinitis in sensitized people.

2. What happens when you have an allergic reaction?

Answer: When a person who is allergic to a particular allergen comes into contact with it, an allergic reaction occurs. This begins when the allergen (for example, pollen) enters the body, triggering an antibody response. The antibodies attach themselves to special cells, called mast cells. When the pollen comes into contact with the antibodies, the mast cells respond by releasing certain substances, one of which is called histamine. When the release of histamine is due to an allergen, the resulting swelling and inflammation is extremely irritating and uncomfortable.

3. What are the most common causes of allergic reaction?

Answer: The most common causes of allergic reactions are:

- dust mites
- pollen (grass, weed or tree)
- foods such as peanuts, cow's milk, soy, seafood and eggs
- cats and other furry or hairy animals such as dogs, horses, rabbits and guinea pigs
- insect stings and tick bites
- molds
- medicines.

Similar reactions can occur to some chemicals and food additives, however if they do not involve the immune system, they are known as "adverse reactions" rather than "allergy."

4. Which areas of body may be mostly affected by an allergic reaction?

Answer: Depending on the allergen and where it enters your body, you may experience different symptoms. For example, pollen, when breathed in through the nose, usually causes symptoms in the nose, eyes, sinuses and throat (allergic rhinitis). Allergy to foods usually causes stomach or bowel problems, and may cause hives (urticaria). Allergic reactions can also involve several parts of the body at the same time.

5. What are the effective treatment options available for treating an allergic reaction?

Answer: Allergen avoidance or minimization relies on identifying the cause of your allergy and then taking steps to reduce your exposure to the allergen. For instance, many people are allergic to dust mites. Therefore reducing dust mite in the house is important. Medications used to treat allergies include Antihistamines, Intranasal corticosteroid nasal sprays (INCS), Adrenaline and various combination therapies. Non-medicated treatments such as saline sprays are used for treating allergic rhinitis and sinusitis. Allergen immunotherapy (also known as desensitization) is a long-term treatment which changes the immune system's response to allergens. It involves the administration of regular, gradually increasing amounts of allergen extracts, by injections or by sublingual tablets, sprays or drops.

6. What are the most reliable allergy tests available?

Answer: Skin prick tests using extracts of allergens and blood RAST or allergen specific IgE tests are most reliable tests for allergic reactions, while as Patch tests are reliable tests for delayed allergic hypersensitivity to chemicals, food and metals.

7. What are the most common allergic diseases?

Answer: The most common allergic diseases are allergic rhinitis, asthma, allergic dermatitis, contact dermatitis, food allergy and urticaria.

8. What is pollen allergy?

Answer: Pollen allergy is an allergic condition affecting the mucous membranes of the nose and the eyes etc., usually characterized by nasal discharge, nasal congestion, and itchy and watery eyes, itchy nose, inner ears and roof of the mouth, that are caused by a hypersensitivity to airborne pollen, such as the pollen of trees, grasses, and weeds.

9. What are the various diseases associated with the occupational allergy reaction?

Answer: The allergic diseases that may be contracted as a consequence of exposure to sensitizing agents in the workplace are rhinitis, conjunctivitis, asthma, eosinophilic bronchitis, hypersensitivity pneumonitis, allergic contact dermatitis, immunologic contact urticaria and occupational anaphylaxis.

10. What are the most common symptoms associated with anaphylaxis?

Answer: Some of the most common symptoms associated with anaphylaxis are:

- Hives, present in 80%-90% of cases
- Nasal congestion, runny nose, itchy eyes.
- Swelling of the tongue and/or throat
- Abdominal discomfort, nausea, vomiting, diarrhea
- Shortness of breath, wheezing, coughing
- Low blood pressure, leading to lightheadedness, passing out, or shock.

11. What are the most reliable allergy tests available?

Answer: Skin prick tests using extracts of allergens and blood RAST or allergen specific IgE tests are most reliable tests for allergic reactions, while as Patch tests are reliable tests for delayed allergic hypersensitivity to chemicals, food and metals.

12. What is anaphylaxis?

Answer: Anaphylaxis is a severe allergic reaction that is potentially fatal. It occurs within minutes of exposure to an allergen. Symptoms include laboured respiration, a precipitous drop in the blood pressure leading to anaphylactic shock followed by contraction of smooth muscles and bronchiolar constriction. This leads to asphyxiation which can lead to death within minutes of exposure to the allergen.

13. What is asthma?

Answer: Asthma is a disease of the bronchial tubes caused by an inflammatory reaction in the lungs following the inhalation of certain substances. In response to a foreign substance, the patient's airways become narrowed, inflamed and filled with excess mucus. Common symptoms include wheezing, coughing, shortness of breath, tightness in the chest, difficulty breathing during or after physical activity.

14. What are the common signs and symptoms seen in hay fever?

Answer: Common symptoms include runny nose and nasal congestion, watery, itchy, red eyes (allergic conjunctivitis), Sneezing, Cough, Itchy nose, fatigue.

15. Can allergies go away on their own?

Answer: Research has shown that allergic reactions can change over time with age and level of exposure, even disappearing in some cases. However, scientists have not been able to explain as to why and how allergies resolve on their own.

ASSIGNMENTS

Q1. Explain the mechanism of pathophysiology of allergic immune response?

Q2. What do you understand by anaphylaxis?

Q3. Explain briefly the various allergies and their effects.

Q4. Describe the preventive measures against aeroallergens.

Q5. Discuss the various diagnostic tests involved in allergy diagnosis.

REFERENCES

Abbas, Abul K, Andrew H. Lichtman, and shiv pillai. *Cellular and molecular immunology.* Philadelphia: saunders/elsevier, 2010. Print.

Barbie D, Mangi A, Lauwers G. Eosinophilic gastroenteritis associated with systemic lupus erythematosus". *J. Clin. Gastroenterol.* 2004 **38** (10): 883–6.

Coico, R. And Sunshine, G. (2015). *Immunology: a short course*. 7th ed. Wiley-blackwell.

Constance Hays, "Ideas & Trends: Airborne Allergies; A New Fear of Flying: Peanuts", *The New York Times* 1998, found at NY Times archives. Accessed March 19, 2009.

Demoly P, Hillaire-Buys D. Classification and epidemiology of hypersensitivity drug reactions. *Immunology and allergy clinics*. 2004 aug 1;24(3):345-56.

Descotes J, Choquet-Kastylevsky G. Gell and coombs's classification: is it still valid? *Toxicology.* 2001 feb 2;158(1-2):43-9.

Jimenez-Saenz M, Villar-Rodriguez J, Torres Y, Carmona I, Salas-Herrero E, Gonzalez-Vilches J, Herrerias-Gutierrez J.. "Biliary tract disease: a rare manifestation of eosinophilic gastroenteritis". *Dig. Dis. Sci.* 2003 **48** (3): 624-7

Kaijser R. Zur Kenntnis der allergischen Affektionen des Verdauugskanals vom Standpunkt des Chirurgen aus. *Arch Klin Chir* 1937; 188:36-64.

Kuby immunology, Judith A Owen; Jenni Punt; sharon a stranford; Patricia P Jones; Janis Kuby, new york: w.h. freeman, ©2013.

Mshra A, Hogan S, Brandt E, Rothenberg M. An etiological role for aeroallergens and eosinophils in experimental esophagitis". *J. Clin. Invest.* 2001 107 (1): 83-90.

Naylor A. Eosinophilic gastroenteritis". *Scottish Medical Journal*. 1990 **35** (6): 163-5.

Passengers with the condition, which can be deadly, can try to ensure a peanut-free flight. But even the best plans sometimes don't work." See "Out of the Blue: Peanut allergies are a little-known danger." Elliott Hester, *St. Petersburg Times*, December 30, 2001, St. Petersburg Times.

Pérez-Millán A, Martín-Lorente J, López-Morante A, Yuguero L, Sáez-Royuela F. Subserosal eosinophilic gastroenteritis treated efficaciously with sodium cromoglycate". *Dig. Dis. Sci*. 1997 42 (2): 342–4.

Perry, T., Conover-Walker, M., Pomes, A., Chapman, M., & Wood, R. Distribution of peanut allergen in the environment." *Journal of Allergy and Clinical Immunology*, 2004 113, 973-76.

Pichler Wj. Drug hypersensitivity reactions: classification and relationship to t-cell activation. *Indrug hypersensitivity* 2007 (pp. 168-189). Karger publishers.

Pringle A, Patek SN, Fischer M, Stolze J, Money NP. The captured launch of a ballistospore". *Mycologia*. 2005 97 (4): 866–71.

Rajan Tv. The gell–coombs classification of hypersensitivity reactions: a re-interpretation. *Trends in immunology*. 2003 jul 1;24(7):376-9.

Riedl Ma, Casillas Am. Adverse drug reactions: types and treatment options. *American family physician*. 2003 nov;68(9):1781-90.

Roitt's essential immunology, Peter J. Delves, Seamus J. Martin, Dennis R. Burton, Ivan M. Roitt. Thirteenth edition. Wiley-blackwell.

The Michael C. Young, M.D., *Common Beliefs About Peanut Allergy: Fact or Fiction?*" Anaphylaxis Canada, 2009.

Trail F. Fungal cannons: explosive spore discharge in the Ascomycota". FEMS Microbiology Letters. 2007. 276 (1): 12–8

Uzzaman A, Cho Sh. Classification of hypersensitivity reactions. In *allergy & asthma proceedings* 2012 may 2 (vol. 33).

Whitaker I, Gulati A, McDaid J, Bugajska-Carr U, Arends M. Eosinophilic gastroenteritis presenting as obstructive jaundice". *European Journal of Gastroenterology & Hepatology*. 2004 16 (4): 407-9.

ABOUT THE EDITOR

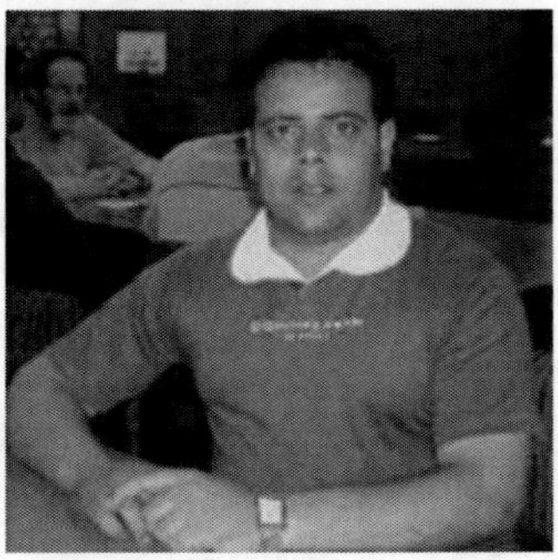

Manzoor Ahmad Mir, JRF-NET, PhD

Senior Assistant Professor, Head Department of Bioresources
School of Biological Sciences, University of Kashmir Srinagar-190006
E-mail: drmanzoor@kashmiruniversity.ac.in

Dr. Manzoor Ahmad Mir holds Master's Degree in Life sciences with Gold medal from HNBG Central University after qualifying prestigious National level CSIR-JRF-NET examination and worked jointly for his Ph. D at Jawaharlal Nehru University New Delhi and CSIR-Institute of Microbial Technology Chandigarh in the field of Immunology and Cell Biology. He currently teaches Endocrinology, Animal Physiology, Immunology and Developmental Biology at the Department of

Bioresources, University of Kashmir, and has been a Research Scientist at SATCAS Stroke Research Chair Majmaah University KSA. Dr Manzoor has research and teaching experience of 13 years and has attended many courses and conferences on immunology, cancer Biology, stroke biology and endocrinology at USA, UK, Kuwait, China, UAE and Saudi Arabia. His basic research interests include molecular immunology, Tuberculosis immunology, Cancer and Stroke Biology. He has published more than 50 high-impact research papers and book chapters, in recognition of which he has received several awards and Royalties from international publishing houses. Dr. Manzoor has authored several books with international publishers like Elsevier USA and Nova Science Publisher USA. He is currently receiving Royalty from Academic Press USA for his book in the field of Immunology entitled “Developing costimulatory molecules for immunotherapy of diseases”. Dr. Manzoor is on the editorial board of some prestigious journals from DOVE medical press New Zealand and Springer Plus UK and has been an invited speaker at various scientific meetings/conferences within India and abroad. He is member of many scientific organizations and societies like International Immunology Association, Indian Association of Immunology, Indian National Science Association, IMMUNOCON etc. Dr Manzoor was awarded Teachers Associate Research Excellence Fellowship (TARE) by DST Govt of India. He has been awarded Summer Research Fellowship Programme (SRFP-2019) by Indian Academy of Sciences and National Science Academy. Dr Manzoor has developed Massive Open Online Course (MOOCs) in Immunology for UG students by sanctioned by UGC- Consortium for Educational Communication (CEC) SWAYAM Ministry of HRD Govt of India. He has been awarded another MOOC Course on Endocrinology by Academic advisory committee of CEC-UGC.

About the Contributors

Umar Mehraj
Junior Research Fellow UGC-CSIR, Research Scholar
Department of Bioresources, School of Biological Sciences,
University of Kashmir Srinagar-190006
E-mail: umarshk92@gmail.com

Safura Nisar
Research Scholar, Department of Bioresources,
School of Biological Sciences, University of Kashmir Srinagar-190006
E-mail: safooranisar99@gmail.com

Hina Qayoom
Research Scholar, Department of Bioresources,
School of Biological Sciences, University of Kashmir Srinagar-190006
E-mail: hinaqkhan1@gmail.com

Syed Suhail
Department of Bioresources, School of Biological Sciences,
University of Kashmir, Srinagar J&K, India

Bashir A. Sheikh
Department of Bioresources, School of Biological Sciences,
University of Kashmir, Srinagar J&K, India

Nissar Ahmad Wani
Department of Biotechnology, School of Life Sciences
Central University of Kashmir, Ganderbal J&K India

INDEX

B

C

E

F

G

H

I

J

K

L

M

N

O

P

Q

R

S

T